Milady's Art and Science of *Nail* TECHNOLOGY

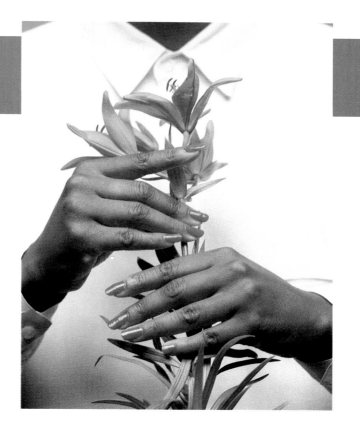

Milady Publishing Company
(A Division of Delmar Publishers Inc.)
2 Computer Dr. W, Box 12519
Albany, NY 12212

CREDITS

Publisher
Catherine Rossbach

Editors
Sheila Furjanic
Jacqueline Flynn

Developmental Editor
Susan Merrill

Project Editor
Judith Boyd Nelson

Production Manager
John Mickelbank

Design Supervisor
Susan C. Mathews

Art Coordinator
Michael Nelson

Art Manager
Rita Stevens

Photo Director
Catherine Frangie

Cover Photographer
Michael A. Gallitelli

Photographer
Michael A. Gallitelli
 on location at the Austin
 Beauty School with
 Deno Petrocelli

Technical Consultant
Tanya Severino

Medical Photographer
Elvin G. Zook, M.D.,
 Division of Plastic Surgery,
 Southern Illinois University
 School of Medicine

Artists
Shizuko Horii
Ron Young

Library of Congress Cataloging-in-Publicaton Data

Milady's art and science of nail technology. — 3rd ed.
    p.   cm.
    Rev. ed. of: The Art and science of manicuring. c1986.
    Includes index.
    ISBN 1-56253-117-4 : (hardcover)—ISBN 1-56253-089-5 (softcover)
    1. Nails (Anatomy)—Care and hygiene. 2. Manicuring. I. Milady
Publishing Company. II. Art and science of manicuring. III. Title:
Art and science of nail technology.
RL94.M48   1992
646.7'27—dc20   91-21945
                                                              CIP

Copyright © 1992
Milady Publishing Company
(A Division of Delmar Publishers Inc.)
2 Computer Dr. W, Box 12519
Albany, NY 12212
   ISBN: 1-56253-117-4 (Hardcover)
           1-56253-089-5 (Softcover)

All Rights Reserved. No part of this work covered by the copyright hereon may be reproduced or used in any form or by any means—graphic, electronic, or mechanical, including photocopying, recording, taping, or information storage and retrieval systems—without written permission of the publisher.

Printed in the United States of America

10 9 8 7 6 5 4 3 2 1

Notice to the Reader

Publisher does not warrant or guarantee any of the products described herein or perform any independent analysis in connection with any of the product information contained herein. Publisher does not assume, and expressly disclaims, any obligation to obtain and include information other than that provided to it by the manufacturer.

The reader is expressly warned to consider and adopt all safety precautions that might be indicated by the activities described herein and to avoid all potential hazards. By following the instructions contained herein, the reader willingly assumes all risks in connection with such instructions.

The publisher makes no representations or warranties of any kind, including but not limited to, the warranties of fitness for particular purpose or merchantability, nor are any such representations implied with respect to the material set forth herein, and the publisher takes no responsibility with respect to such material. The publisher shall not be liable for any special, consequential or exemplary damages resulting, in whole or in part, from the readers' use of, or reliance upon, this material.

Contents

PREFACE ix

ACKNOWLEDGMENTS xii

INTRODUCTION 1

PART I GETTING STARTED

Chapter 1
YOUR PROFESSIONAL IMAGE 6
Introduction 7
Professional Salon Conduct 7
• Professional Salon Conduct Toward Clients 7
• Professional Salon Conduct Toward Employers and Coworkers . 9
Professional Ethics 10
• Professional Ethics Toward Clients 10
• Professional Ethics Toward Employer and Coworkers 11
Your Professional Appearance 12

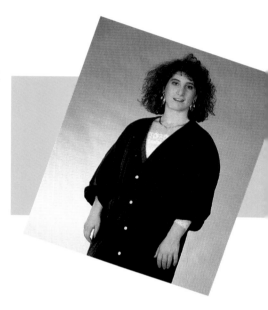

Chapter 2
BACTERIA AND OTHER INFECTIOUS AGENTS 14
Introduction 15
Bacteria 15
• Types of Bacteria 15
• Growth and Reproduction of Bacteria 17
• Movement of Bacteria 17
Viruses 17
• Acquired Immune Deficiency Syndrome (AIDS) 17
Fungus and Mold 18
• Nail Fungus 18
• Nail Mold 18
Parasites 19
Rickettsia 19
Understanding Infection 19
• Immunity to Infection 19
• How Infections Breed in the Salon 20
• How Nail Technicians Can Fight Infections 21

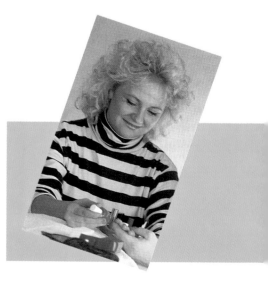

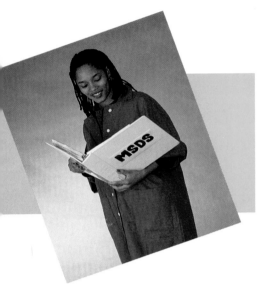

Chapter 3
SANITATION 23
Introduction 24
Methods of Sanitation 24
• Sanitation with Physical Agents 25
• Sanitation with Chemical Agents 25
• Equipment Used in Sanitation 25
• Chemical Sanitizing Agents 27
• What is an Approved Disinfectant? 28
• Pre-Service Sanitation Procedure 29
• End-of-Day Sanitation 31
Safety Precautions 31

Chapter 4
SAFETY IN THE SALON 32
Introduction 33
Common Chemicals Used by Nail Technicians 33
Learn About the Chemicals in Your Products 34
• What is an MSDS? 34
How Products Can Harm You 35
How to Protect Yourself and Your Clients 36

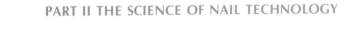
PART II THE SCIENCE OF NAIL TECHNOLOGY

Chapter 5
ANATOMY AND PHYSIOLOGY 40
Introduction 41
Cells 41
• Cell Growth 42
• Cell Metabolism 42
Tissues 43
Organs 43
Systems 44
The Skeletal System 44
• Structure of Bone 45
• Joints 45
• Bones of the Arm and Hand 45
• Bones of the Leg and Foot 46
The Muscular System 47
• Muscle Parts 48
• Stimulation of Muscles 49
• Muscles Affected by Massage 49
The Nervous System 52
• The Brain and Spinal Cord 52
• Nerve Cells and Nerves 53
The Circulatory System 55
• The Heart 55
• The Blood 56

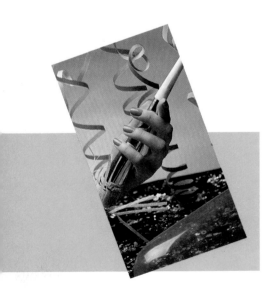

The Endocrine System 59
The Excretory System 59
The Respiratory System 60
The Digestive System 60

Chapter 6
THE NAIL AND ITS DISORDERS 62
Introduction 63
Parts of the Nail 63
• Parts of the Nail 63
• Structures Beneath the Nail 63
• Skin Surrounding the Nail 64
Nail Disorders 64
• Nail Disorders That Can be Serviced by a Nail Technician 65
• Nail Disorders That Cannot be Serviced by a Nail Technician ... 69

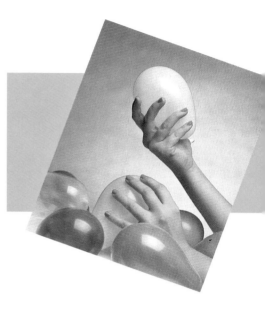

Chapter 7
THE SKIN AND ITS DISORDERS 72
Introduction 73
Healthy Skin 73
• Function of the Skin 73
• Structure of the Skin 74
• Nourishment of the Skin 76
• Nerves of the Skin 76
• Glands of the Skin 77
• Elasticity of the Skin 78
Skin Disorders 78
• Lesions of the Skin 79
• Inflammations of the Skin 80
• Infections of the Skin 81
Pigmentation of the Skin 81
Hypertrophies (New Growths) of the Skin 82

Chapter 8
CLIENT CONSULTATION 83
Introduction 84
Determining the Condition of Nails and Skin 84
Determining Your Client's Needs 85
Meeting Your Client's Needs 85
Completing the Client Health/Record Card 86
Maintaining the Client Service Record 89

PART III BASIC PROCEDURES

Chapter 9
MANICURING 92
Introduction 93
Nail Technology Supplies 93
• Equipment 93
• Implements 94
• Materials 96
• Nail Cosmetics 97

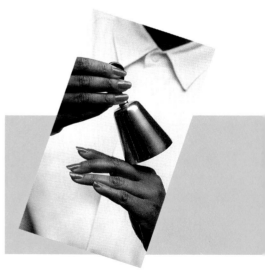

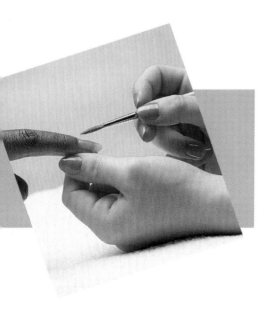

Procedure for Basic Table Set-Up 100
Choosing a Nail Shape 101
Water Manicure 102
• Water Manicure Pre-Service 102
• Water Manicure Procedure 103
• Water Manicure Post-Service 108
French Manicure 109
Reconditioning Hot Oil Manicure 109
• Supplies 110
• Reconditioning Hot Oil Manicure Pre-Service 110
• Reconditioning Hot Oil Manicure Procedure 110
Man's Manicure 111
• Procedure 111
Electric Manicure 115
Hand and Arm Massage 116
• Hand Massage Techniques 116
• Arm Massage Techniques 117

Chapter 10
PEDICURING 120
Introduction 121
Supplies 121
Pedicure 122
• Pedicure Pre-Service 122
• Pedicure Procedure 123
• Pedicure Post-Service 126
Foot Massage 127
• Foot Massage Techniques 127

PART IV THE ART OF NAIL TECHNOLOGY

Chapter 11
NAIL TIPS 132
Introduction 133
Supplies 133
Nail Tip Application 134
• Nail Tip Pre-Service 134
• Nail Tip Procedure 134
• Nail Tip Post-Service 137
Maintenance and Removal of Tips 138
• Maintenance 138
• Tip Removal 138

Chapter 12
NAIL WRAPS 140
Introduction 141
Fabric Wraps 141
• Supplies 141
• Nail Wrap Pre-Service 141
• Nail Wrap Procedure 142
• Nail Wrap Post-Service 144

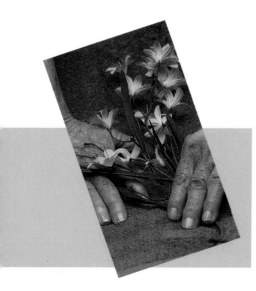

Fabric Wrap Maintenance, Removal, and Repairs 145
• Fabric Wrap Maintenance.....................................145
• Repairs with Fabric Wraps 147
• Fabric Wrap Removal 147
Paper Wraps 148
• Supplies 148
Paper Wrap Application Procedure 148
Liquid Nail Wrap 149

Chapter 13
ACRYLIC NAILS...151
Introduction 152
Acrylic Nails over Forms 152
• Supplies 152
• Acrylic Nail Pre-Service 153
• Acrylic Nail Procedure 153
• Acrylic Nail Post-Service 157
Acrylic Nails over Tips or Natural Nails........................158
• Procedure 158
Acrylic Nails over Bitten Nails 160
• Procedure 160
Acrylic Nail Maintenance and Removal 162
• Acrylic Maintenance..162
• Acrylic Removal 165
Odorless Acrylics 166

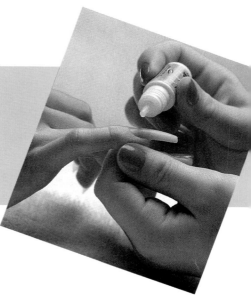

Chapter 14
THE CREATIVE TOUCH 168
Introduction 169
Light-Cured Gel on Tips or Natural Nails 169
• Supplies 169
• Gel Application Pre-Service 170
• Light-Cured Gel Procedure 170
• Gel Application Post-Service 172
Light-Cured Gel over Forms 172
No-Light Gel Application 174
Gel Maintenance and Removal 175
• Gel Maintenance..175
• Gel Removal 175
Creating Nail Art 176
• Gems 176
• Striping Tape 176
• Foil 177
• Procedure for Holly Berries 178
• Procedure for "The Sweep" 179
• Procedure for Marbled Gold 179
• Using an Air Brush 180

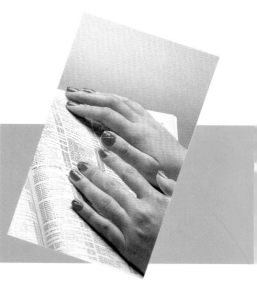

PART V THE BUSINESS OF NAIL TECHNOLOGY

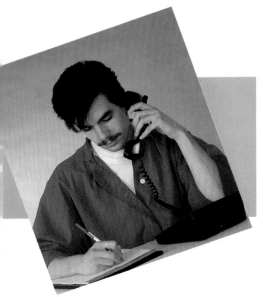

Chapter 15
SALON BUSINESS 182
Introduction 183
Your Working Environment 183
• The Full-Service Salon 183
• The Nails-Only Salon 183
• Making Your Decision 184
Keeping Good Personal Records 185
• Income 185
• Expenses 185
• Appointments 185
Understanding Salon Business Records 186
• Using Business Records 186
• Keeping Client Records 187
• Keeping Inventory Records 187
Booking Appointments 187
Advertising Yourself 189
Collecting Payment for Services 189

Chapter 16
SELLING NAIL PRODUCTS AND SERVICES 190
Introduction 191
Know Your Products and Services 191
• Features 191
• Benefits 192
Know What Your Client Needs and Wants 192
Present Your Products and Services 193
• Sell While You Work 193
• Display a List of Your Services 193
• Display Your Products 193
Answer Questions and Objections 194
• Questions 194
• Objections 194
Close the Sale 195
• Suggestion Selling 195
• Wrap-Up 195
• Scheduling Another Appointment 195

ANSWERS TO REVIEW QUESTIONS 196

GLOSSARY/INDEX 217

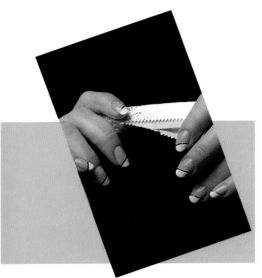

Preface

Nail technology is an exciting and rewarding profession. Each year professional nail technicians perform more than $3 billion worth of manicuring, pedicuring, and artificial nail services for millions of fashion-conscious clients.

Milady's Art and Science of Nail Technology, third edition, is the complete guide to basic nail technology that every professional nail technician has been waiting for. It is more than a revision of our popular basic manicuring text, *The Art and Science of Manicuring*, second edition, by Alice Cimaglia. Two-thirds of the content in the third edition is **entirely new material**.

When the staff at Milady began the revision process, we surveyed **you**, the users of the book. Through hundreds of surveys, formal focus groups, and detailed written critiques, you told us what you wanted in a new nail technology book, **and we listened**.

FEATURES OF THIS EDITION

In response to **your needs**, this exciting new edition of *The Art and Science of Nail Technology* includes the following features:

- **Chapters and Parts.** The book is divided into sixteen chapters and five parts so it is much easier to use.

- **Full-Color Art.** All art is in **full color**, with actual photographs to show you step-by-step procedures for manicuring, pedicuring, tips, wraps, acrylic nails, and basic nail art procedures.

- **Learning Objectives and Review Questions.** Learning objectives provide goals for the students in each chapter. These objectives are reinforced by review questions that assess how well the student has mastered the goals established in the learning objectives. The answers to these review questions are conveniently located at the back of the book. They can be used by students to study for exams.

- **Actual Photos of Nail Disorders**. For the first time in any nail technology or cosmetology book, full-color photos are included to help students identify nail disorders more accurately.

- **Client Consultation Guidelines.** A complete chapter focuses on client consultation and gives suggestions for identifying and meeting the needs of each individual client.
- **Chemical Safety Coverage.** A complete chapter is devoted to the important topic of chemical safety in the nail salon. Students will learn to identify the chemicals commonly used in the nail salon, how they can cause harm, how to protect themselves and their clients, and how to read an MSDS (Material Safety Data Sheet).
- **State Licensing Exam Topics.** The topics required for state licensing examinations are presented in a complete, easy-to-read fashion.
- **Safety Cautions.** Highlighted safety cautions alert students to services that include potentially dangerous procedures. These cautions explain how to avoid dangerous situations and how to provide services in a safe, clean environment.
- **Sanitation Cautions.** Highlighted sanitation cautions give specific suggestions for maintaining proper sanitation at all times.
- **Procedural Tips.** Procedural tips provide hints on the most efficient and effective way to complete step-by-step procedures. These tips help students improve their nail technology skills.
- **State Regulation Alerts.** Because state regulations vary, state regulation alerts remind students to check with their instructors for specific regulations in their state.

SUPPLEMENTS FOR THE STUDENT AND INSTRUCTOR

The *Art and Science of Nail Technology*, third edition, features three entirely new supplements:

Milady's Nail Technology Workbook

This workbook is a valuable student supplement that coordinates chapter-by-chapter with the textbook. It strengthens the students' understanding of nail technology by reinforcing the material covered in the textbook. The workbook includes short answer, short essay, sentence completion, matching, definition, labeling, and word review activities. The workbook also includes a final exam review made up of multiple choice questions and a series of situational tests that ask students what they would do in a difficult situation if they were the nail technician.

Answers to Milady's Nail Technology Workbook

This is an easy-to-use teacher's edition of the workbook that provides answers for all workbook questions and activities.

Milady's Nail Technology Course Management Guide

This step-by-step, simple-to-use course guide has been designed specifically to help the nail technology instructor set up and operate a successful nail technology training program. It includes:

- Guidelines for starting and implementing a nail technology program
- Detailed lesson plans for each chapter in the book
- Handouts ready for use in the classroom
- Transparency masters for easy-to-create visual aids
- A Chemical Safety Program that can be implemented in the nail technology classroom

Acknowledgments

The staff of Milady Publishing Company wishes to acknowledge the many individuals and organizations who helped shape this edition of Milady's Art and Science of Nail Technology. Their input enabled us to produce a book that will be a valuable resource for both students and professionals in the field of nail technology. To all those who contributed to this edition we extend our sincere thanks and appreciation.

- Barbara Abramovitch
New England Hair Academy
Malden, MA

- Suzanne Arduini
Albany, NY

- Jan Austin
Austin Beauty School
Albany, NY

- Giselle Bohamde
Austin Beauty School
Albany, NY

- Dale Bona
C.H. McCann Vocational
Technical High School
North Adams, MA

- Jason Boulla
Albany, NY

- Bich Ly
Albany, NY

- Burmax Co.
Hauppauge, NY

- Patricia Castro
College of San Mateo
San Mateo, CA

- Alice Ciurlino
P & B Beauty School
Gloucester, NJ

- Deborah Clark
Albany, NY

- Elizabeth Coleman
Albany, NY

- Howard Conlon
Bellaire Beauty College
Bellaire, TX

- Suzanne Council
Van Michael Salon
Atlanta, GA

- Van Council
Van Michael Salon
Atlanta, GA

- Matthew Creo
Autsin Beauty School
Albany, NY

- Nancy Court
Arnold Beauty College, Inc.
Fremont, CA

- Wilma Curry
Bellaire Beauty College
Bellaire, TX

- Brenda De Angelo
Daytona Beauty School
Daytona Beach, FL

- Arnold DeMille
Milady Publishing Consultant
Continuing Education Specialist
New York, NY

- Christine DeRusso
Albany, NY

ACKNOWLEDGMENTS   xiii

- Peggy Dietrich
Laredo Beauty College
Laredo, TX

- Luciano Di Paolo
Euclidian Beauty College Inc.
Euclid, OH

- Barbara Dorsey
Baltimore Stud. of Hair Design
Baltimore, MD

- Cindy Drummy
Nails Magazine
Redondo Beach, CA

- Carol Duffy
Alameda Beauty College
Alameda, CA

- Roslyn Duncan
Debbie's School of Beauty Culture
Houston, TX

- Dana Ennello
Mechanicville, NY

- Barbara Feiner
NailPro Magazine
Van Nuys, CA

- Flo Finch
Northland Pioneer College
Holbrook, AZ

- Marion Ford
Albany, NY

- Laverne Foster
Pat Goins Beauty Schools
Monroe, LA

- Nehme Frangie
Albany, NY

- Jamal Frangie
Albany, NY

- Wadad Frangie
Austin Beauty School
Albany, NY

- Anne Fretto
Stanton, CA

- Nancy Gallitelli
Albany, NY

- Ray Gambrell
South Carolina State Board of Cosmetology
Greenwood, SC

- Anthony Gardy
Albany, NY

- Sharon Gill
Garden State Academy
South Bound Brook, NJ

- Cynthia Gimenez
Arnold Beauty Colleges, Inc.
Remont, CA

- Anne Golloway
Ossining, NY

- Aurie Gosnell
National Interstate Council of Cosmetology
Aiken, SC

- Constance Gregg
Boca Raton Institute
Boca Raton, FL

- Ann Harrell
St. Petersburg, FL

- Linda Harris
Maxims Beauty Academy
Blaine, MN

- Danielle Hasberry
Albany, NY

- Helen Heine
South Eastern College of Beauty Culture
Charlotte, NC

- Michael Hill
Arkansas State Board of Cosmetology
Fayetteville, AR

- Frances Hoffman
Manatee Area Vocational Technical Center
Bradenton, FL

- Barbara Hogue
Arizona Academy of Beauty
Tucson, AZ

- Linda Howe
Pittsburgh Beauty Academy
Pittsburgh, PA

- Sally Hudson
Tampa Bay Career Academy
Tampa, FL

- Karen Iolli
Ailano School of Cosmetology
Brockton, MA

- Frank Jacobi
Citrus Community College
Glendara, CA

- Janice Jaynes
Institute of Cosmetology
Houston, TX

- Julia Jefferson
Vogue College of Hair Design
Highland Heights, KY

- Dorothy Johnson
Yuma School of Beauty
Yuma, AZ

- Spring Kelsey
Earlton, NY

- Glenn Kewley
Drome Sound Music Store
Schenectady, NY

- Paulette Know
Antioch Beauty
Antioch, CA

- L. Jean Lake
Elaine Steven Beauty College
St. Louis, MO

- Carol Laubach
San Jacinto College
Pasadena, TX

- Denise Leach
Oakland Technical Center
South East Campus
Royal Oak, MI

- Inna Lozhkin
Albany, NY

- Charles Lynch
International Beauty School
Lancaster, PA

- Tina Macki
Albany, NY

- Laura Manicho
Nationwide Beauty Academy
Cols, OH

- Sharon Matern
Albany, NY

- Patricia Mc Daniel
Bellaire Beauty College
Bellaire, TX

- John Mickelbank
Albany, NY

- Louise Miller
Lamson Academy of Hair Design
Phoenix, AZ

- Ruth Miller
Quincy Beauty Academy
Quincy, MA

- Marcia Miller
Federico Beauty College
Fresno, CA

- Pauline Moram
Innerstate Beauty School
Bedford Heights, OH

- Mary Ann Morris
House of Heavilin
Blue Springs, MO

- Eileen Morrissey
Maison de Paris Beauty College
Haddon Field, NJ

- Florence Nebblett
Washington, DC

- Neka Beauty Supplies
Albany, NY

- Pat Nix
Indiana State Board of Cosmetology
Booneville, IN

- Theda O'Brien
Albany, NY

- John Olsen
Phagan's Beauty School, NW
Tigard, OR

- Susan Peters
Lansdale School of Cosmetology
Lansdale, PA

- Dino Petrocelli
Albany, NY

- Nilsene Privette
College of Beauty and Art and Science
Sedona, AZ

- Lois Purewal
Spring Branch Beauty College
Houston, TX

- Irma Quezada
Pipo Academy of Hair Design
El Paso, TX

- Sarah Rainey
St. Augustine Technical Center
St. Augustine, FL

- Jennifer Rhatigan
Albany, NY

- Cleolis Richardson
Philadelphia, PA

- Jim Rogers
Milpitas Beauty College
Milpitas, CA

- Betty Romesberg
The Head Hunters
Cuyahoga Falls, OH

- Richard Scher, MD
College of Physicians and Surgeons
Columbia University
New York, NY

- Douglas Schoon
Chemical Awareness Training Service
Irvine, CA

- Regina Schrenko
Northhampton, PA

- Joan Sesock
Austin Beauty School
Albany, NY

- Tanya Severino
Albany, NY

- Sandra Skoney
Toledo Academy of Beauty Culture
Toledo, OH

- Jenny Smith
Vogue Beauty College
Idaho Falls, ID

- Alicia Solazzo
Bronxville, NY

- Bertha Stanko
Menands, NY

- Judith Stewart
PJ's College of Cosmetology
Carmel, IN

- Alma Tilghman
North Carolina Board of Cosmetology
Beaufort, NC

- Sandy Tirpak
Albany, NY

- Mona Townsend
Backscratchers Nail Care Products
Sacramento, CA

- Wendy Trainor
Schuylerville, NY

- Veda Traylor
Arkansas State Board of Cosmetology
Mayflower, AR

- Barbara Turman
School of Nail Technology Inc.
Coral Gables, FL

- Peggy Turbyfill
Mike's Barber and Beauty Salon
Hot Springs, AR

- Beverly Venable
Loudonville, NY

- Judy Ventura
Dudley Cosmetology University
Kernersville, NC

- Dave Welsh
J & D Supply
Albany, NY

- Renee Wilson
Argyle, NY

- Lois Wiskur
South Dakota Cosmetology Commission
Pierre, SD

- Victoria Wurdinger
New York, NY

- Jack Yahm
Milady Publishing Consultant Emeritis
"Father of Cosmetology Accreditation"
Lauderdale Lakes, FL

- Linda Zizzo
Milwaukee Area Technical College
Milwaukee, WI

- Elvin Zook, M.D.
Southern Illinois University School of Medicine
Springfield, IL

The Milady staff would like to thank the following individuals and organizations for their assistance:

For the use of photographs:

Salon on pages 2 and 183 courtesy of
Takara Belmont U.S.A., Inc.
Harvey Allen Salon
Merrick, NY
(Award of Special Distinction,
Modern Salon of the Year Award, 1991)
Thomas Stanwood, Photographer

Manufacturer's representative on page 2 courtesy of
Backscratchers Nail Care Products Inc.

Model on page 2 courtesy of
OPI Products, Inc.
Nail Fashion by OPI International Design Team

Salon manicuring area on page 183 courtesy of
Takara Belmont U.S.A., Inc.
Urban Retreat
Houston, Texas
(Grand Prize, Modern Salon of the Year Award, 1991)
James F. Wilson, Photographer

Photographs of onycholysis caused by trauma and onycholysis on page 70 courtesy of
Orivlle J. Stone, M.D.
Dermatology Medical Group
Huntington Beach, California
and NAILS Magazine

For help with supplies:

Carl J. Mione
Vice President/School Sales
Burmax
Hauppauge, NY 11788

Neka Beauty Supplies
Albany, New York

OPI Products, Inc.

Dave Welsh
J & D Supply
Albany, New York
(Safety glasses)

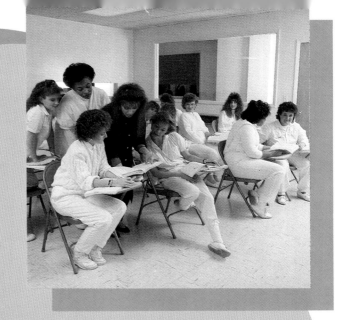

Introduction

Introduction

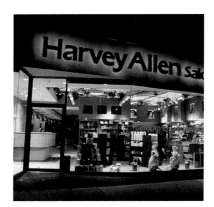

Welcome to the exciting world of nail technology.

You have chosen to become a nail technician, one of the fastest-growing and most creative, rewarding, and high-paying professions in cosmetology today. As a nail technician you will use the latest technology to apply artificial nails. You will use your artistic abilities to create original designs on nails. Your work will be relaxed and comfortable, with many successful and fashionable clients, some of whom may pay as much as $125 an hour for a service. You will be part of the booming manicuring, pedicuring, and artificial nail industry, with combined sales of more than $3 billion a year. This figure represents more than a 25 percent increase over previous years in some areas, and continues to climb.

Because nail technology is a complex, changing profession you will want to continue learning even after you receive a license. You may start your career as a nail technician in a salon. As you develop your knowledge and skills, you may want to move into other career areas in nail technology. These careers include teaching nail technology in cosmetology schools or demonstrating manufacturer's nail products at shows, conventions, or stores. You can become a salon owner or even the personal nail technician for fashion models or actors on the stage, in movies, or on TV. You can write, edit, or be a consultant for nail technology books and magazines.

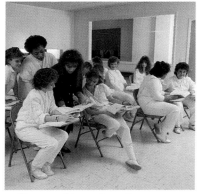

You could teach nail technology.

Nail technology has changed in the 5000 years since the first manicure was recorded. Manicures used to be a luxury enjoyed only by rulers and the wealthy, and were performed by servants. Today, nail technology is enjoyed by millions of fashion-conscious people from many social and economic groups. In most states today nail technology services are performed by licensed professionals who have completed up to 500 hours of classroom instruction. During instruction they learn to improve the health of their clients'

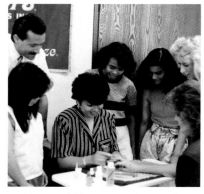

You could be a manufacturer's representative.

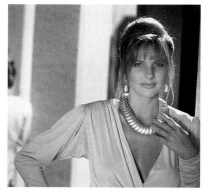

You could be a personal nail technician for a fashion model.

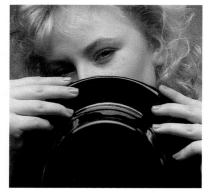

You could be a nail technician for actors in the theater.

nails and recognize healthy nails and skin, as well as possible nail and skin disorders. They become skilled in using the latest nail technology while following proper sanitation and safety procedures to protect both themselves and their clients. Today's professional nail technicians learn how to give pedicures to enhance the look of their clients' feet, improve health, and relieve stress. They also learn how to handle the business aspects of their profession.

The first manicures did not require formal instruction. The word "manicure" comes from the Latin "manus" (hand) and "cura" (care). The first evidence of nail care recorded in history was before 3000 BC in Egypt and China. Ancient Egyptian men and women of high social rank stained their nails with a red-orange dye called henna, which comes from a shrub. The color of a person's nails in ancient Egypt was a sign of importance. Kings and queens wore deep red, while people of lower rank were allowed to wear only pale colors. Around 3000 BC the Chinese developed a nail paint made from beeswax, egg whites, gelatin, and gum arabic. In 600 BC, Chinese royalty wore gold and silver paint on their nails. In the 15th Century, leaders of the Chinese Ming Dynasty painted their nails black and red. Military commanders in Egypt, Babylon, and early Rome spent hours before a battle having their hair lacquered and curled and their nails painted the same shade as their lips.

As a 20th Century nail technician, you can give your clients many more choices for nail care than the privileged people of ancient civilizations had. You can offer your clients a basic manicure or pedicure and information about nail care. They can also choose from a variety of artificial nail services shaped, colored, and designed specifically to their needs. You will become a successful nail technician by studying hard and learning the skills and professional manner to make all your clients feel like 20th Century kings and queens. Let's get started studying this exciting field.

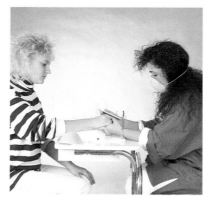

You will learn proper sanitation and safety procedures.

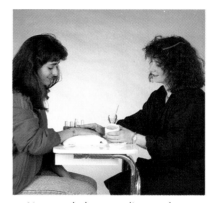

You can help your clients select the products and services that meet their needs.

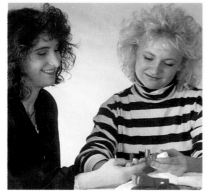

You can offer your clients a variety of nail technology services.

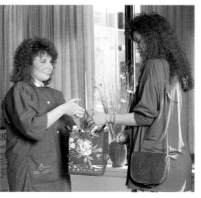

You can use your skills to build a steady, happy clientele.

PART I

GETTING STARTED

- *Chapter 1 - Your Professional Image*
- *Chapter 2 - Bacteria and Other Infectious Agents*
- *Chapter 3 - Sanitation*
- *Chapter 4 - Safety in the Salon*

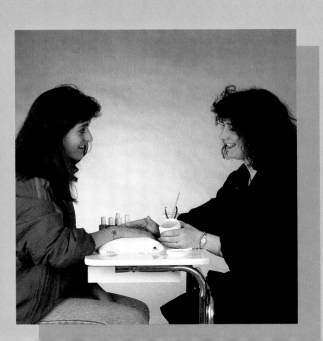

CHAPTER 1

Your Professional Image

LEARNING OBJECTIVES

After you have studied this chapter, you should be able to:
1. Define salon conduct.
2. Give examples of professional salon conduct toward clients.
3. Give examples of professional salon conduct toward employers and coworkers.
4. Define professional ethics.
5. Give examples of professional ethics toward clients.
6. Give examples of professional ethics toward employers and coworkers.
7. Describe the type of appearance you should have as a professional nail technician.

Introduction

When you are a successful nail technician you will be able to do more than give an expert manicure, create natural-looking artificial nails, or paint original designs on a client's nail. You will know how to behave in a professional manner. You will follow the rules for professional behavior with clients, employers, and coworkers. You will also develop good personal health and grooming habits. In this chapter, you will learn the rules of professionalism for nail technicians. They include proper salon conduct, professional ethics, and how to present yourself to clients as an attractive and well-groomed representative of the nail technology industry. If you practice these rules, you will quickly build a satisfied clientele that will lead to your success.

Professional Salon Conduct

Salon conduct is the way you behave when you are working with clients, your employer, and coworkers in a salon.

PROFESSIONAL SALON CONDUCT TOWARD CLIENTS

Set high standards for proper salon conduct. You can create an environment in your salon that is relaxed and pleasant for clients and makes them want to come back and bring their friends.

1. **Be on time.** You will appear relaxed, competent, and concerned about your clients' needs if you are on time, waiting to serve them when they arrive. Being late can make you seem disorganized or uncaring. It is discourteous and can annoy and inconvenience your clients.

2. **Be prepared.** Before your clients arrive, make sure your station is completely set up with an adequate supply of materials and equipment. Make sure your implements are sanitary and ready to use.

3. **Plan your day.** Keep an appointment schedule near you for each day so that you know what you are supposed to do every hour. The schedule should include your client's name, service to be performed, time of appointment, and client's phone number. Call your clients by name when they arrive. When you know what service you are to perform, you can begin without hesitation and give your clients a feeling of security. (Fig. 1.1)

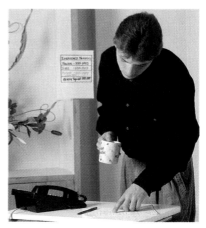

1.1 — Plan your day carefully.

4. **Arrange appointments carefully.** Schedule your appointments so that each client has enough time. If you schedule too many clients during your day, you won't have time to serve them and some will have to wait or be rescheduled for another day. If the receptionist makes appointments for you, be sure to give him or her a neat list of the services you offer and the time you need to complete each one.

5. **Keep clients informed of schedule changes.** Contact clients if your appointments are running very late or if you have to reschedule their appointments. They will appreciate your honesty and they will be grateful that you haven't wasted their time.

6. **Be courteous.** Have a cheerful, friendly, and helpful attitude. This attitude will tell your clients that you care for them. Before you perform any service, you can make your clients feel comfortable and relaxed. Help them take off their coats and show them where to sit for the service. All new clients can be given a tour of the salon and shown where the rest rooms and phones are. You may also tell them how to book future appointments, how to reschedule an appointment, and what forms of payment your salon accepts.

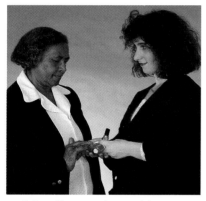

1.2 — Communicate with your client.

7. **Perform all tasks willingly and efficiently.** Never make your clients feel their appointments inconvenience you.

8. **Communicate with your clients.** Explain the services you will perform for your clients and the retail products needed to maintain these services. Listen to their concerns with undivided attention and answer their questions. No matter how successful you become, always keep your attitude humble when dealing with your clients. (Fig. 1.2)

9. **Never complain to, or argue with, a client.** Try to keep any conversation on a professional level at all times. While you are performing nail services, you can use the time to explain what you are doing and why. You can also suggest and discuss other salon services or products that could help your client.

10. **Use good judgment.** Do not share information about your personal life or personal stories about other clients, your coworkers, or your employer with your client. Concentrate on your client's needs.

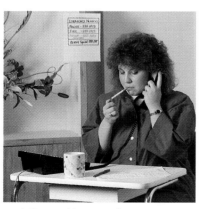

1.3 — Never chew gum, smoke, or eat where you can be seen by clients.

11. **Never chew gum, smoke, or eat where you can be seen by clients.** These habits can be extremely annoying to clients and smoking can be dangerous around nail chemicals. (Fig. 1.3)

PROFESSIONAL SALON CONDUCT TOWARD EMPLOYERS AND COWORKERS

It is important to work closely with your employer and coworkers because it will help create a strong, successful salon that will eventually secure your future in this industry. To be competitive, the entire staff must work together. You want to create an atmosphere that will make your clients enjoy their visits to your salon so much they will not want to go to another.

Below are guidelines to follow for dealing with employers and coworkers.

1. **Communicate.** Establish an open, honest line of communication between yourself and your employer. Be perfectly honest about your strengths and weaknesses. Make sure your work meets the standards the salon expects.

2. **Be willing to learn.** Keep an open mind and be willing to accept suggestions. Don't automatically assume that your way of doing something is the only correct way. Nail products and services are improved often; be prepared to update your skills.

3. **Give credit to others.** Never take credit for another person's ideas. Try to acknowledge contributions made by others.

4. **Respect the opinions of coworkers.** Your ideas and opinions are important, but yours are not the only ones. Frequently, the ideas of many people create the best solution.

5. **Take the initiative.** Never be afraid to offer help or suggestions to make things better or easier for your employer or coworkers.

6. **Use good judgment.** If you have a problem or question about your job, discuss it directly with your employer, not with your clients or coworkers.

7. **Leave personal problems at home.** Do not tell your personal problems to your employer, fellow employees, or clients. Personal problems are distractions that interrupt the concentration needed to do a good job.

8. **Never borrow money from employers or coworkers.** This is a practice that can result in a very awkward work situation. Eventually your coworkers may lose respect for you.

9. **Promote the salon.** Learn about the other services offered at your salon, such as hair care, skin care, and cosmetic consultations so you can promote the entire salon to clients.

10. **Develop your ability to sell.** Explain the benefits of products and services to clients without pressuring them.

Professional Ethics

Professional *ethics* (**ETH**-iks) is your sense of right and wrong when you interact with your clients, employer, and coworkers. The essential values in professional ethics are honesty, fairness, courtesy, and respect for the feelings and rights of others.

PROFESSIONAL ETHICS TOWARD CLIENTS

High ethical standards for treating clients will earn you a good reputation. Your clients will trust you, keep coming back, and bring their friends. Your best source of advertising is through the recommendations of clients who respect and trust you.

1. **Suggest services that meet your clients' needs.** Never suggest or give clients services they don't need or want, or ones that could harm them. Explain what you recommend for your clients and why, so they will feel comfortable with your services.
2. **Keep your word and fulfill all obligations.** Always do what you have promised the client and what the client wants you to do. Don't take short cuts because you are rushed or substitute other services because they are more convenient for you.
3. **Treat all your clients fairly.** Never offer special discounts or services to one client and not to another.
4. **Follow your state regulations for sanitation and safety.** Always follow provisions of the state laws covering nail technology. Regulations may seem inconvenient at times, but they are created to protect you and your clients. To be an ethical nail technician, you must always be knowledgeable about current laws concerning your profession.
5. **Be loyal.** Never complain, gossip, or talk to your client about other clients, your employer, or coworkers. Your clients will not trust you if you talk about other people to them because they will think you will talk about them the same way.
6. **Don't criticize others.** Never criticize the services offered by other nail technicians or other salons. Even if the client insists on discussing another colleague's or salon's service, you may listen, but remain neutral in your responses.
7. **Don't abandon your clients.** If you leave the manicuring field or move to another community, give your clients enough notice to find another nail technician or recommend a coworker or colleague you trust. If you have a large clientele, consider training someone to take your place. You want your clients to experience the least amount of discomfort.

Nails First

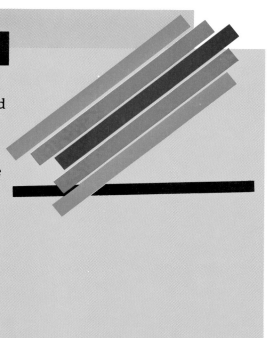

Nothing promotes your business more than the appearance of your own nails. Clean, neatly trimmed nails and healthy cuticles build your business; chipped and uneven nails erode client confidence. How can you keep your nails neat through hours of daily use? To protect your nails while you work, use gloves whenever your hands come in contact with primers, liquid bonders, or other chemicals. Slather hand lotion on before you slip the gloves on, and they'll seal in the lotion and help it penetrate. To avoid chipping your polish, keep nails highly buffed or coated with clear polish only. Never use the free edge of your nail to remove polish from the client's cuticle. A cotton-tipped orangewood stick dipped in polish remover will do the job and save your nails.

PROFESSIONAL ETHICS TOWARD EMPLOYER AND COWORKERS

By using professional ethics to support the efforts and morale of your coworkers and employers, you will help contribute to the success of your salon. As the salon becomes more successful, so will you.

1. **Be honest.** Never blame a coworker for your mistakes. Take responsibility for your own actions.

2. **Fulfill your obligations.** Keep any promises you make to an employer or coworker, such as coming in on your day off to help with a special client. If you cannot possibly keep a promise, contact your employer or coworker ahead of time and ask if you can help to make other arrangements.

3. **Respect the talents of your employer and coworkers.** Praise them and encourage them when they do a good job. Try not to criticize.

4. **Don't invite criticism of coworkers.** When you hear a client complain about another technician, do not take sides. You don't know all the facts and it is not your business. Suggest that the client speak directly to the coworker involved. Never

criticize someone else's work. Let your standards and work speak for themselves. If another's work is exceptionally poor, offer to repair your client's nails without placing blame on another nail technician.
5. **Never gossip or start rumors among coworkers.** Some people think these tactics can get them ahead in business, but they only serve to make you look bad and alienate your associates.

Your Professional Appearance

You should be a model of good grooming for your clients because you are a member of the beauty industry. Your clients expect you to look your best. You should be pleasant to be around. You must be clean and pleasant-smelling so clients will not object to having you touch them while you perform nail services. They should find it pleasant to sit across from you while you perform nail services. (Fig. 1.4)

1. **Be clean and fresh.** Bathe or shower daily and use an effective deodorant.
2. **Have fresh breath and healthy teeth.** Make sure your breath is fresh at all times. Do not eat garlic or spicy foods that can give you bad breath during the working day. Keep a toothbrush, toothpaste, and mints with you so you can freshen your breath when needed. Keep your teeth and gums healthy by regular brushing and dental check-ups.
3. **Wear clean clothes that are appropriate for the salon.** Always wear clean, pressed clothes to the salon. You should look your best in stylish, comfortable clothes, but not be overdressed. (Fig. 1.5)
4. **Pay attention to your hair, skin, and nails.** Make sure your hair is neat, you have on just enough make-up to enhance your natural beauty, and your nails are well-manicured.

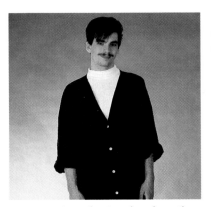

1.4 — A professional male nail technician

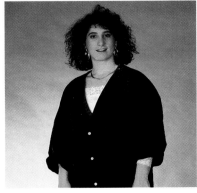

1.5 — A professional female nail technician

Review Questions

1. What is salon conduct?
2. Give ten examples of professional salon conduct toward clients.
3. Explain why a salon might lose clients if nail technicians do not exhibit professional salon conduct.
4. Give ten examples of professional salon conduct toward employers and coworkers.
5. Define professional ethics.
6. Give seven examples of professional ethics toward clients.
7. Give five examples of professional ethics toward employers and coworkers.
8. Describe the type of appearance you should have as a professional nail technician.
9. Explain why a salon might lose clients if it employs nail technicians who have an unprofessional appearance.

CHAPTER 2

Bacteria and Other Infectious Agents

LEARNING OBJECTIVES

After you have studied this chapter, you should be able to:
1. *Define bacteria and describe their appearance.*
2. *Explain the difference between pathogenic and non-pathogenic bacteria.*
3. *Identify the main groups of pathogenic bacteria and describe each of them.*
4. *Name and describe the types of cocci.*
5. *Describe the process of mitosis and explain why it is important to bacterial growth.*
6. *Give examples of common infections caused by viruses.*
7. *Explain how it is possible to transfer AIDS in the salon.*
8. *Describe the appearance of nail mold at its various stages of development.*
9. *Name the different types of immunity.*
10. *Name the common sources of infection in the salon.*
11. *Explain the ways that nail technicians can fight infections within the salon.*

Introduction

The nail technician's job is not usually thought to be a dangerous one, but without proper sanitation, both you and your clients are in great danger of infection from bacteria, viruses, fungi, mold, and parasites. The kinds of infections that can be transmitted during nail services range from the common boil, to fungus that can cause the loss of a nail, to the life-threatening AIDS virus. When you learn what infection is and how it is spread, you will be better prepared to prevent it with proper sanitation procedures.

Bacteria

Bacteria (bak-**TEER**-ee-ah) are one-celled vegetable *microorganisms* (meye-kroh-**OR**-gah-niz-ems) so small they can only be seen through a microscope. Fifteen hundred of them barely cover the head of a pin. A single gram of soil can contain as many as 2.5 billion bacteria. Bacteria are the most plentiful organism on earth. There are 15,000 known species of bacteria, and they can exist nearly everywhere. They multiply at an incredible speed. A single bacterial cell can produce 16,000,000 more in only half a day.

Bacteria are found in water, air, dust, lint, and decaying matter. They are on the skin of the body, in the secretions of body openings, on clothing, on your manicuring table, on your implements, and under nails.

TYPES OF BACTERIA

Bacteria are classified into two types, depending on whether they are beneficial or harmful.

1. **Nonpathogenic** (non-path-o-**JEN**-ik) (non-disease-causing) bacteria can't harm us and are often beneficial. About 70 percent of all bacteria are nonpathogenic. These bacteria play the important role in nature of *decomposing* (de-kom-**POH**-zing) or breaking down matter. They belong to the *saprophyte* (**SAP**-ro-fyt) group of bacteria that feed on dead matter and cause decay. Some forms of nonpathogenic bacteria help produce food and oxygen. Others are used in compost piles to improve the fertility of the soil.

    In humans, nonpathogenic bacteria are most numerous in the mouth and intestines, where they help the digestive process by breaking down food.
2. **Pathogenic** (path-o-**JEN**-ik) (disease-causing) bacteria are harmful. Though less than 30 percent of all bacteria are pathogenic, bacteria are the most common cause of infection

and disease in humans. Pathogenic bacteria are also called *microbes* or *germs*. They invade living plant or animal tissues and feed on living matter. They breed rapidly and spread disease by producing *toxins,* or poisons, in the tissue they invade.

Classification of Pathogenic Bacteria

There are three main groups of pathogenic bacteria. They include:

1. *Cocci* (**KOK**-si). These are round, pus-producing bacteria. Cocci appear singly or in groups as follows: (Fig. 2.1)

    a) **Staphylococci** (staf-i-lo-**KOK**-si) grow in clusters and are present in local infections, such as abscesses, pustules, and boils. (Fig. 2.2)

    b) **Streptococci** (strep-to-**KOK**-si) grow in chains. They cause strep throat and infections or diseases that spread throughout the body such as blood poisoning and rheumatic fever. (Fig. 2.3)

    c) **Diplococci** (deye-ploh-**KOK**-si) grow in pairs and cause pneumonia. (Fig. 2.4)

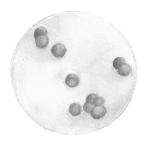

2.1 — Cocci

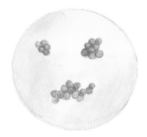

2.2 — Staphylococci

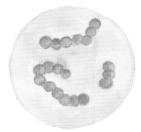

2.3 — Streptococci

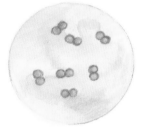

2.4 — Diplococci

2. *Bacilli* (bah-**SIL**-i). These are the most common bacteria. They are rod-shaped and produce such diseases as tetanus, influenza, typhoid, tuberculosis, and diphtheria. (Fig. 2.5)

3. *Spirilla* (spi-**RIL**-a). These are spiral or corkscrew-shaped bacteria that include spirochetal organisms. One example of these bacteria is treponema pallida (trep-o-**NE**-mah **PAL**-i-dah), which causes syphilis. (Fig. 2.6)

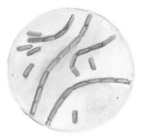

2.5 — Bacilli

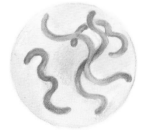

2.6 — Spirilla

GROWTH AND REPRODUCTION OF BACTERIA

Bacteria live, grow, and multiply best in warm, dark, damp, unsanitary conditions. The drawer of your manicuring table is a perfect place to breed bacteria on unsanitized implements.

Each bacterium, or bacteria cell, has the ability to grow and reproduce. As bacteria are nourished, each bacterium cell grows in size. When it reaches maturity, it divides crosswise into halves and forms two identical cells. This division is called mitosis (meye-**TOH**-sus). The cells continue to grow until they are mature and divide, forming four cells. One bacterium can reproduce into as many as 16 million bacteria in 12 hours.

When conditions become unfavorable for growth and reproduction, many types of bacteria form a tough outer covering called a spore. Then they remain dormant, or in a state of rest. Bacteria, such as anthrax and tetanus, can survive periods of famine, dryness, and unsuitable temperature. In this stage, the spore can be blown about in the dust and is not harmed by disinfectants, heat, or cold. When conditions become favorable, they again begin to grow and reproduce. (See Chapter 5, page 42, for more information on mitosis.)

MOVEMENT OF BACTERIA

Bacteria travel very easily. They are spread through air or water, or through contact with contaminated objects. Bacilli and spirilla are the only bacteria that can propel themselves. They have hairlike projections known as *flagella* (flah-**JEL**-ah) or *cilia* (**SIL**-ee-a), which they move in a whiplike motion to propel themselves in liquid.

Viruses

Viruses are pathogenic (disease-causing) agents that are many times smaller than bacteria. Viruses enter a healthy cell, grow to maturity, and reproduce, often destroying the cell. Hepatitis, chicken pox, influenza, measles, mumps, and the common cold are examples of viral infections that can be transferred through casual contact with an infected person. Infection spreads when the person sneezes or coughs.

ACQUIRED IMMUNE DEFICIENCY SYNDROME (AIDS)

Acquired Immune Deficiency Syndrome (AIDS) is a disease caused by the HIV virus. AIDS attacks and eventually destroys the body's immune system. The disease may lie dormant in an infected person's system for up to 10 years, but it can mature into a fatal disease in 2 to 10 years.

Unlike most other viruses, HIV cannot be transferred through casual contact with an infected person, sneezing, or coughing. AIDS is passed from one person to another through the transfer of bodily fluids such as semen and blood. The most common methods of transferring AIDS are through (a) sexual contact with an infected person, (b) the use of dirty hypodermic needles for intravenous drug use, (c) the transfusion of infected blood. AIDS can also be transferred from mother to child during pregnancy and birth.

It is possible to transfer AIDS in the salon through the use of unsanitized manicuring implements. If you were to nip the cuticles of a client infected with AIDS you might transfer blood to your cuticle nippers. Then if you nipped another client and transferred the AIDS infected blood to the second client, that client might get AIDS.

Fungus and Mold

Fungi (**FUN**-gi) is the general term for vegetable *parasites* including all types of fungus and mold. The types of concern to the nail salon are nail fungus and nail mold. Both are contagious. They can spread from nail to nail on the client and from the client to the nail technician.

NAIL FUNGUS

Nail fungus usually appears as a discoloration in the nail that spreads toward the cuticle. As the condition matures, the discoloration becomes darker. Fungus may affect the hands, feet, and nails. Clients with nail fungus must be referred to a physician. (Fig. 2.7)

NAIL MOLD

Nail mold is a type of fungus infection caused when moisture is trapped between an unsanitized natural nail and products that are put over the natural nail, such as tips, wraps, gels, or acrylic nail products.

Nail mold can be identified in the early stages as a yellow-green spot that becomes darker in advanced stages. If the nail has been infected for a period of time, the discoloration becomes black and the nail softens and smells bad. If these conditions exist, the nail will probably fall off.

Exposing the Natural Nail

You should not provide nail services for a client who has nail fungus or nail mold, but the client may want you to remove any artificial nail covering to expose the natural nail. After the natural nail is exposed, the client should be referred to a physician.

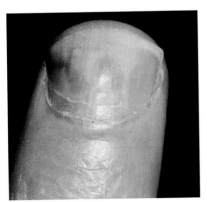

2.7 — Nail fungus (mold)

You should wear gloves during removal of artificial nails and follow the manufacturer's directions for removal. When the artificial nail has been removed, discard orangewood sticks, abrasives, and any other porous product used. Completely sanitize all other implements, linen, and the table surface before and after the procedure.

Prevention

Nail mold and fungus may be avoided by following sanitary precautions. Do not perform nail services for a client who has discoloration on his or her nails. Do not take short cuts or omit any of the sanitation steps when performing an artificial nail service.

Parasites

Parasites (**PAR**-ah-syts) are multicelled animal or vegetable organisms. They live off living matter without providing any benefits to their hosts. An example of vegetable parasite infection is ringworm. Animal parasites are responsible for such contagious diseases as scabies, itch-mite, and pediculosis (lice).

Rickettsia

Rickettsia (rik-**ET**-see-ah) are much smaller organisms than bacteria, but larger than viruses. They cause typhus and Rocky Mountain spotted fever. Fleas, ticks, and lice carry rickettsia.

Understanding Infection

An *infection* occurs when body tissue is invaded by disease-causing microorganisms such as bacteria, viruses, and fungi. Microorganisms establish themselves and multiply in body tissue to produce tissue damage. At first, the infection is usually localized. If the infection spreads to the bloodstream and it carries toxins to all the parts of the body, it is called a general infection. Blood poisoning is a type of general infection.

IMMUNITY TO INFECTION

All living organisms have defenses or immunity against infection. *Immunity* (i-**MYOO**-ni-tee) is the ability of the body to resist disease and destroy microorganisms when they have entered the body. Immunity against disease is a sign of good health. Immunity can be natural, naturally acquired, or artifically acquired.

immunity. By keeping our bodies healthy, we are able off microorganisms before they can grow and cause . Our bodies fight infection in three ways.

have a protective layer of unbroken skin.

naturally secrete perspiration and digestive juices that courage the growth of disease-causing microorganisms.

ur blood contains white corpuscles and *antitoxins* that ll germs and counteract the poisons produced by them.

urally acquired immunity. After fighting off a disease, ibodies, a type of protein molecule, remain in the bloodeam ready to fight another attack of the microorganisms at caused that disease.

rtificially acquired immunity. This immunity is one produced y the injection of a serum or vaccine that introduces a small dose of disease-causing microorganism into the body. This small dose stimulates the body's growth of antibodies that can fight that disease.

HOW INFECTIONS BREED IN THE SALON

Most bacteria, viruses, fungi, and other disease-causing germs enter the body through the nose, the mouth, and small breaks in the skin. They can also enter your body through your eyes or ears.

You are at risk of becoming infected or transmitting infection to your clients because you come in constant contact with germs in the salon. Some of the common sources of infections include:

1. **Contaminated manicuring tools and equipment.** Bacteria and other germs multiply at a very rapid rate in places such as dirty nail files, cuticle nippers, manicuring tables, and towels. (Fig. 2.8)

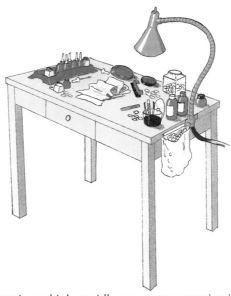

2.8 — Bacteria multiply rapidly on a messy manicuring table.

2. **Your clients' nails, hands, and feet.** E̶ walks into the salon brings in a whole new ⟨ you perform a service on this client, you ri̶ by these germs. When you perform artificial na̶ risk trapping your clients' germs between her nat̶ and the artificial nail.

3. **Your clients, coworkers, and your own mouth, nose, an̶** Anyone in the salon who has a cough, is sneezing, or h̶ runny nose is like a fountain of germs.

4. **Open wounds or sores on you or your client.** Infected fluids can be transferred from one person to another through open wounds.

5. **Objects throughout the entire salon.** Germs collect on chairs, tables, towels, bottles, brushes, and everything else that is exposed to the air in the salon. They also collect on the fixtures in the restroom—especially the door handle.

HOW NAIL TECHNICIANS CAN FIGHT INFECTIONS

You are responsible for keeping yourself and your clients safe from infection. Here are the steps to take:

1. **Learn proper sanitation procedures and follow them.** Chapter 3 in this book describes the procedures to follow for proper sanitation. It is your responsibility to yourself and your clients to learn proper sanitation procedures and follow them faithfully. If you decide to short-cut sanitation procedures, you could easily become infected or transmit infection to your clients.

2. **Do not work in contagious conditions.** You should not work with clients while they are *contagious* (kon-**TAY**-jus), or have an infection that can easily be transmitted from one person to another. Someone with a severe cold, influenza, or chicken pox, for example, should not receive nail services. You should also stay home and rest if you are contagious because it is very easy to pass infection to your clients.

3. **Do not work near an open wound.** Refer any client who has an open wound to a physician.

4. **Do not cause wounds.** Be very careful when you are performing nail services. It is easy to nip a client while you are nipping cuticles or to break the skin if you file too deeply.

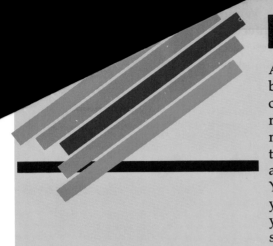

Capturing Clients During Cutbacks

Are cutbacks in client income cutting into your client base? Some salons are attracting budget-conscious clients by offering a special discount program. One night a week, clients are invited to visit the salon for nail services at a special, lower price—and there's no tipping. The atmosphere is festive, with lively music and refreshments. What's in it for the nail technicians? Your satisfied client on bargain night might become your steady client during regular salon hours. And if you need to perfect your skills on a special nail service, here's your chance because there are no appointments and the salon manager can match nail technicians with clients. You can ask for clients who want fiberglass wraps, gel nails, or whatever service you want to perfect. What's in it for the salon? On a busy night a salon can make up for lower prices by servicing more cleints.

Review Questions

1. What are bacteria? What do bacteria look like?
2. Are all bacteria harmful? Give examples to explain your answer.
3. What are the three main groups of pathogenic bacteria? Describe each of them.
4. Name and describe three types of cocci.
5. Describe the process of mitosis. Explain why it is important to bacterial growth.
6. Give examples of common infections caused by viruses.
7. Explain how it is possible to transfer AIDS in the salon.
8. Describe the appearance of nail mold at its various stages of development.
9. What is immunity? Name three types of immunity.
10. Name five common sources of infection in the salon.
11. Explain four ways that you can fight infections within the salon.

CHAPTER 3

Sanitation

LEARNING OBJECTIVES

After you have studied this chapter, you should be able to:
1. Describe the difference between sterilization and sanitation.
2. Identify the different methods of sanitation.
3. List the types of equipment used to sanitize.
4. Name the different methods of sanitizing with physical agents.
5. Explain why sterilization is impractical in a salon.
6. List the safety precautions to follow when using chemical agents for sanitation.

Introduction

When you become a nail technician, you will be licensed to touch, massage, and apply potentially harmful chemicals to the hands, feet, and nails of the general public. Whenever you work with the public there is the danger of infection or injury to you and to your clients. This danger exists if your implements and work area are not properly sanitized or you do not use sanitizing chemicals properly. Because infections and some diseases can be spread through the type of physical contact nail technicians have with clients, states have strict rules for sanitation procedures at manicuring work stations. In this chapter, you will learn proper sanitation procedures to enable you to pass state licensing exams and become a licensed nail technician. Proper sanitation will help protect you against possible lawsuits from clients who have become injured or infected during your nail service.

> **STATE REGULATION ALERT**
>
> *You must obey the rules issued by your local Health Department and your state cosmetology regulatory agency. Be alert for changes in the rules and regulations in your area. For your own safety and that of your clients, it is extremely important that you obtain and obey sanitation rules and regulations.*

Your work station and implements must be sanitized, not sterilized, to meet state health requirements. *Sterilize* means to make something germ-free by destroying all bacteria. *Sanitize* means to make something clean and prevent germs from growing on it. Sanitized areas are not germ-free. Health departments and state cosmetology regulatory agencies know it is possible to have a sterile area only if it is sealed off from everything like air and human contact. Sterilization is impractical in a salon. But, you must sanitize your area and equipment.

The term "sanitize" will be used to indicate all forms of sanitation in this chapter.

Methods of Sanitation

There are two methods of sanitation:

- Sanitation that uses *physical agents* such as ultraviolet rays, moist heat, and dry heat.
- Sanitation that uses *chemical agents* such as alcohol, quats, and formalin.

SANITATION WITH PHYSICAL AGENTS

Physical sanitation agents include ultraviolet rays, moist heat, and dry heat.

Ultraviolet rays

Most bacteria are killed or weakened by exposure for more than two to three hours to invisible light rays in this method of sanitation. Salons and schools put implements in electrical sanitizers that use ultraviolet rays to kill bacteria. Since ultraviolet radiation is harmful to eyes, you must shield your eyes from exposure.

Moist heat

Two moist-heat methods of sanitation are used — boiling and steaming. *Boiling* destroys bacteria at 212° F or 100° C, the boiling points for water. This method is not practical in the salon because it is slow and can damage equipment and implements, especially plastic.

To destroy bacteria by *steaming* you need a piece of equipment called an autoclave. An *autoclave* uses steam pressure to sanitize. This machine is not practical for salons because it is expensive and inconvenient.

Dry heat

Bacteria are killed by exposure to intense heat or baking. This method is used in hospitals.

SANITATION WITH CHEMICAL AGENTS

Chemicals are the most effective and easy-to-use sanitizing agents. They include antiseptics and disinfectants.

An *antiseptic* (an-ti-**SEP**-tik) is usually a liquid that may kill or retard the growth of bacteria. Antiseptics are safe to use on clients' feet, hands, and nails. They are not strong enough to sanitize your implements.

A *disinfectant* (dis-in-**FEK**-tant) is stronger than an antiseptic. It cannot be used on skin, and it is strong enough to sanitize implements. A fumigant (**FYUM**-i-gant) is a kind of disinfectant. It is used with a dry or cabinet sanitizer.

Some chemicals can be classified as either antiseptic or disinfectant depending on their strength. For example, quaternary compounds, or "quats" can be mixed in a strong solution and be considered a disinfectant. They can also be mixed in a weaker solution, with more water, and be considered an antiseptic.

EQUIPMENT USED IN SANITATION

There are three types of equipment used to sanitize. They are wet sanitizer, dry/cabinet sanitizer, and ultraviolet sanitizer.

1. *Wet sanitizer.* Any glass receptacle that is large enough to hold disinfectant solution and a submerged, or completely covered implement, can be used as a wet sanitizer. Wet sanitizers have

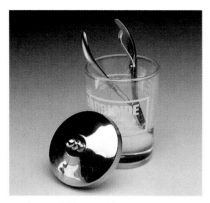

3.1 — Wet sanitizer

a cover to prevent contamination of the disinfectant. When implements are dry, they should be put in a dry/cabinet sanitizer or a completely sanitized and sealed box, cabinet, or drawer until they are used. (Fig. 3.1)

2. *Dry/cabinet sanitizer.* A dry or cabinet sanitizer is an airtight cabinet in which you place formaldehyde (for-**MAL**-de-heyed) tablets which will produce an active fumigant. It is possible to buy formaldehyde gas but the tablets are safer because they are premeasured. Sanitized implements are stored in sanitary conditions by keeping them in the cabinet until ready to use. Formaldehyde gas has a strong odor and caution must be taken when it is being used. Replace chemicals every two days because they lose strength in that time.

3. *Ultraviolet ray electrical sanitizer.* This type of sanitizer is also used to keep implements clean until ready for use. Implements must be sanitized before they are placed in the ultraviolet sanitizer. Follow manufacturer's directions for proper use.

How to Make Percentage Sanitizing Solutions with Chemical Agents

You may be able to buy chemical sanitizing agents in the strengths required by your state. However, you should know the formulas for preparing different strengths of chemical sanitizing solutions. The following formulas are for solutions that are called percentage solutions because they contain a percentage of chemical agent. The higher the percentage, the stronger the solution. For example, a 70 percent alcohol solution is 70 percent alcohol and 30 percent water; a 90 percent alcohol solution is 90 percent alcohol and 10 percent water. The chart below gives you formulas for the different solutions in U.S. units and metric units. Each state may require different strength solutions for sanitizing.

Solution %	Chemical Agent	Water
1%	3/4 tsp.	12 oz.
	6 ml	500 ml
2%	1 1/2 tsp.	12 oz.
	11 ml	500 ml
4%	3 tsp.	12 oz.
	21 ml	500 ml
5%	4 tsp.	27 ml
	27 ml	500 ml
10%	8 tsp.	12 oz.
	56 ml	500 ml
20%	6 tbl.	12 oz.
	125 ml	500 ml

Solution %	Chemical Agent	Water
25%	1/2 c.	12 oz.
	167 ml	500 ml
50%	1 1/2 c.	12 oz.
	500 ml	500 ml
70%	3 1/2 c.	12 oz.
	1167 ml	500 ml
90%	3 1/2 qts.	12 oz.
	4500 ml	500 ml

CHEMICAL SANITIZING AGENTS

Quaternary Ammonium Compounds (Quats)

Quaternary ammonium (**QUAT**-er-nery a-**MOHN**-ee-um) *compounds* include a broad range of chemical agents. Quats are available under different trade and chemical names and come in liquid and tablet form. They are part of products you will use as disinfectants, cleansers, sterilizers, and fungicides for sanitation.

The advantages of quats as a sanitation agent are that they are odorless, colorless, non-toxic, and stable. The disadvantage is that they may not be effective sanitizing agents against the HIV virus.

A 1:1000 solution of quats is commonly used to sanitize implements. Immersion time is at least 20 minutes.

How to Prepare a 1:1000 Strength Solution of a Quaternary Ammonium Compound

If the chemical contains:

10 percent active ingredient, add 1¼ oz. (37.5 ml) quat solution to 1 gallon (3.8 l) of water.

12½ percent active ingredient, add 1 oz. (30 ml) quat solution to 1 gallon (3.8 l) of water.

15 percent active ingredient, add ¾ oz (22.5 ml) quat solution to 1 gallon (3.8 l) of water.

Formalin

Formalin (**FOHR**-mah-lin) is an effective sanitizing agent used as a disinfectant. Formalin is approximately 37 percent to 40 percent of formaldehyde gas in water when purchased. Formalin should be used with great care because inhalation can cause damage to mucous membranes and contact with the skin can cause irritation. Because of its potential danger, formalin is most commonly added to prepared sanitizing agents in various strengths, as follows:

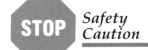

Safety Caution

Do not breathe formalin or allow it to come in contact with your skin. It can damage your mucous membranes and cause skin irritation.

25 percent Solution (equivalent to 10 percent formaldehyde). Used to sanitize implements. Immerse them in the solution for at least 20 minutes. (Preparation: 2 parts formalin, 5 parts water, 1 part glycerine to prevent rust.)

10 percent Solution (equivalent to 4 percent formaldehyde). Used to sanitize combs and brushes. Immerse them for at least 20 minutes. (Preparation: 1 part formalin, 9 parts water.)

Sanitation with Alcohol

To sanitize **manicuring** or other **implements**, immerse them in 70 or 90 percent alcohol for 20 or more minutes.

Sanitation with Sodium Hypochlorite

Salon owners have added *sodium hypochlorite* (**SOH**-di-um hy-po-**CHLOR**-ite) compounds to the list of sanitizing agents they use because of the threat of the HIV virus. It can be used to sanitize your implements but can be very corrosive to metal implements. The pure compound, common household bleach, can be used also. Manicuring implements should be immersed in a 10 percent solution of sodium hypochlorite for 10 or more minutes.

WHAT IS AN APPROVED DISINFECTANT?

The chart below will help you use the sanitizing agents that are approved in your state.

Chemical Agent	Form	Strength	How to Use
Quaternary ammonium compounds	Liquid or tablet	1:1000 solution	Immerse implements in solution for 20 or more minutes.
Formalin	Liquid	25% solution	Immerse implements in solution for 10 or more minutes.
Formalin	Liquid	10% solution	Immerse implements in solution for 20 or more minutes.
Alcohol	Liquid	70% or 90% solution	Immerse implements for 20 or more minutes.
Sodium hypochlorite (household bleach)	Liquid	10% solution	Immerse implements in solution for 10 or more minutes.

STATE REGULATION ALERT

Consult your state cosmetology regulatory agency or the Health Department for a list of approved disinfectants in your state.

PRE-SERVICE SANITATION PROCEDURE

1. **Wash implements.** Wash implements thoroughly with soap and warm water.

2. **Rinse implements in plain water.** Rinse all traces of soap with plain water. Dry thoroughly with a sanitary towel.

3. **Immerse implements in wet sanitizer.** Immerse implements in wet sanitizer containing an approved disinfectant for the required time (usually 20 minutes). (Fig. 3.2)

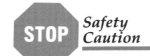 **Safety Caution**

Check the disinfectant solution in your wet sanitizer after each client. If it is cloudy, the solution is contaminated and must be replaced.

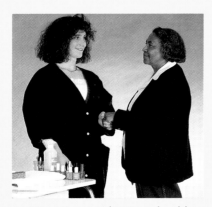

3.2 — Your workstation should be completely sanitized when your client arrives.

4. **Wash hands with antibacterial soap.** Thoroughly wash your hands with antibacterial soap, rinse, and dry with sanitized towel.

5. **Rinse implements and dry with sanitary towel.** Remove implements from wet sanitizer, rinse in water, and wipe dry with clean towel to prevent rusting.

PROCEDURAL TIP

▶ *It is a good idea to have two sets of manicuring implements because it takes 20 minutes for them to be sanitized in the wet sanitizer.*

6. **Follow approved storage procedure.** Follow your state regulations for storage of sanitized manicuring implements. The regulations will tell you to store sanitized implements in sealed containers, sealed plastic bags, or to keep them in cabinet sanitizer until ready to be used.
7. **Disinfect table.** Wipe manicuring table with disinfectant solution.
8. **Wrap client's cushion in clean towel.** Put a clean towel over your manicuring cushion. Be sure to use a clean towel for each client.
9. **Refill disposable materials.** Put new emery board, orangewood stick, cotton balls, and other disposable materials on manicuring table. These materials are discarded after use on *one* client.

PROCEDURAL TIP

▶ *After each procedure that involves artificial nails, discard your plastic trash bag. This will prevent the release of fumes from products you've used.*

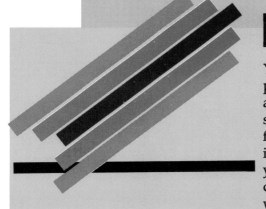

Order Seafood and a Salad for Your Nails

You can help your clients maintain healthy nails by passing along some basic information about vitamins and minerals. To keep their nails healthy, clients should eat foods high in calcium (dairy products and fish); sulphur (cabbage, onions, garlic, and cucumber); iodine (seafood); iron (spinach, apricots, grapes, egg yolk, and green vegetables); vitamin A (watercress, dandelion, carrots, tomatoes, apricots, melon, and wheat germ); vitamin B (wheat germ, liver, cabbage, celery, and fish); vitamin C (tomatoes, lemons, oranges, grapefruit, and cabbage); and vitamin D (fish, liver, and mushrooms). Your clients will appreciate the good advice and your work will appear that much nicer on strong, healthy nails.

END-OF-DAY SANITATION

At the end of the day perform a final sanitation procedure on your work area, implements, and equipment. Store implements in one of the sanitary environments mentioned above.

Safety Precautions

The use of chemical agents for sanitation involves certain dangers, unless safety measures are taken to prevent mistakes and accidents.

1. Purchase chemicals in small quantities and store them in a cool, dry place; otherwise, they deteriorate upon contact with air, light, and heat.
2. Weigh and measure chemicals carefully.
3. Keep all containers labeled and stored under lock and key.
4. Do not smell chemicals or solutions, as many of them have pungent odors and can cause lung damage.
5. Avoid spilling when dissolving or diluting chemicals.
6. If you accidentally spill a chemical agent on your clothing, remove the soiled garment immediately.
7. Keep a complete first aid kit on hand.
8. Follow manufacturer's directions.
9. Be sure to watch small children at your work station. A child can accidentally spill or ingest chemicals without proper supervision.

Review Questions

1. What is the difference between sterilization and sanitation?
2. Describe the two methods of sanitation.
3. List three types of equipment used to sanitize.
4. What are four different ways to sanitize with physical agents?
5. Why isn't sterilization practical in a salon?
6. What are three safety precautions to follow when using chemical agents for sanitation?

CHAPTER 4

Safety in the Salon

LEARNING OBJECTIVES

After you have studied this chapter, you should be able to:
1. *Identify the chemicals commonly used by nail technicians.*
2. *List the early warning signs of overexposure to nail chemicals.*
3. *Describe what an MSDS is.*
4. *Define flashpoint.*
5. *Explain how products can enter the body and cause harm.*
6. *Identify ways you can protect yourself and your clients when using chemicals in the salon.*

Introduction

Today anyone can have long, beautiful nails thanks to the advances of chemistry and the scientific and artistic talents of nail technicians. We can make short nails long, long nails strong, and we can turn anyone's nails into a work of art.

Most nail technicians are skilled in services such as nail tips, nail wraps, acrylic nails, and gel nails. For each of these services you will use "hi-tech" chemicals that could harm both you and your clients. None of the products you use every day as a nail technician *need* to harm your health, but all of them *can*.

You will learn step-by-step procedures for giving your clients advanced nail services in Chapters 11-14. But first, in this chapter, you will learn some basic rules for using nail chemicals safely and wisely.

Common Chemicals Used by Nail Technicians

If you perform advanced nail services, your manicuring table is full of chemical products including:

- Nail polish and nail polish remover that both contain solvents
- Liquid and powder for acrylic nails
- Primer for acrylic nails
- Gel nail supplies for both light-cured and no-light gels
- Adhesive dryer (or gel activator)
- Glue for fabric wraps

You shouldn't be afraid of these chemicals. Exposure to them won't harm you, but *overexposure* is a danger you need to avoid.

How can you tell if you have been overexposed? Your body will give you signs. The most common early warning signs of overexposure to nail chemicals include the following problems:

- Light-headedness
- Insomnia
- Runny nose
- Sore, dry throat
- Watery eyes
- Tingling toes
- Tiredness all day
- Irritability
- Sluggishness
- Breathing problems

Learn About the Chemicals in Your Products

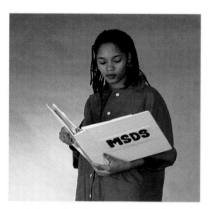

4.1 — Read your MSDS sheets.

Manufacturers, for the most part, do a good job of making products as safe as possible. But they can only do so much. Many of their positive efforts can be undone by a single careless act by a nail technician. It's up to you to learn about the chemicals in your products and how to handle them safely.

One excellent way to learn about the potential hazards, proper handling, and signs of overexposure for any product is by reading the Material Safety Data Sheet (MSDS) for that product. (Fig. 4.1)

WHAT IS AN MSDS?

The United States government requires that product manufacturers make *Material Safety Data Sheets* available to people who work with their products. Each MSDS must contain twelve basic items of information. There is no standard form for manufacturers to use in writing an MSDS, but all of the following information must be included:

1. **Identity of chemicals presenting physical or chemical hazards.** This information may not be very specific if manufacturers have received an exemption because of trade secret provisions.

2. **Physical and chemical characteristics.** This section will include the product's *flashpoint* (the temperature at which a liquid will give off enough flammable vapor to ignite).

3. **Physical hazards.** How this product reacts with other chemicals, potential for explosion, and fire hazards.

4. **Health hazards.** General signs and symptoms of illness that might be caused by this product and existing medical conditions that might be aggravated by this product.

5. **Primary routes of entry into the body.** How the chemical usually enters your body.

6. **Permissible exposure limits.** Recommended limits to prevent overexposure.

7. **Carcinogen hazard of the chemical.** Information about whether the product can cause cancer.

8. **Precautions and handling procedures.** How to handle the product safely and what to do if it leaks or spills.

9. **Control and protection measures.** How to protect yourself and clients against the hazards of the product. Suggested ventilation, glove usage, safety glass usage, protective clothing, and protective equipment.

10. **Emergency and first aid procedures.** How to handle accidents while using the product.

11. **Preparation date.** When the MSDS was prepared and updated or changed.

12. **Writer.** Name, address, and phone number of the person who was responsible for preparing the MSDS.

How You Can Get Material Safety Data Sheets

Your local distributor of beauty supplies should be able to supply you with MSDSs for the products that you buy from them. It is your responsibility to collect these sheets and keep them available for reference. If you have difficulty collecting the MSDSs you need, send a formal written request to the distributor.

How Products Can Harm You

Although MSDSs will provide you with specific information about any product you're using, there is some general information you should know. Products enter your body in three ways:

- You breathe them (*inhalation*).
- You absorb them through your skin (*skin contact*).
- You eat them (*ingestion*).

But products don't have to enter your body to harm you. Some are flammable. Others can seriously damage you if they splash or fly into your eyes.

A few examples of potential health and safety problems are:
- Solvents and primers can cause serious injury if they come in contact with your eyes. Each time you sit down to do nails, you could lose your vision if you're not extremely careful.
- It's unhealthy to breathe the dust created when you file acrylic nails and vapors from acrylic products, solvents, and primers.
- Nail polish and nail polish removers are extremely flammable.
- Etching primers are extremely corrosive to skin.
- Wrap glues, acrylic liquids, gels, and solvents dry your skin and cause it to crack and peel. Chemicals can enter your body through broken skin.

How to Protect Yourself and Your Clients

You can protect both yourself and your clients if you follow some very important safety rules:

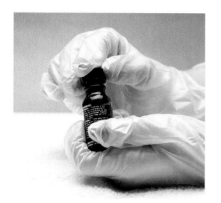

4.2 — Wear gloves when using primer.

1. **Ventilate.** Work in a ventilated salon. It's important that your ventilation system remove vapors from the building instead of just circulating them around the salon. This means that the system has to be vented to the outside. Vented manicuring tables are somewhat effective, but the charcoal filters fill up every 20 hours. If the filters aren't changed, the vented tables no longer do their job.

2. **Avoid spraying products into the air.** It's easier to keep vapors out of the air if you use drop-on or brush-on products. If drop-on or brush-on products aren't available, choose pumps over aerosols.

3. **Keep products off of skin.** Wear gloves when using strong chemicals, especially primer, and try to keep products off of both your skin and your client's skin. Barrier creams can slow down the rate at which your skin absorbs chemicals, but they *aren't* invisible gloves. Invest in a supply of latex or rubber gloves and be sure to dispose of them when they become contaminated. (Fig. 4.2)

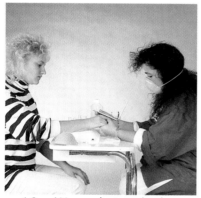

4.3 — Wear a dust mask when filing and offer one to your client.

4. **Wear a dust (surgical) mask when you're filing.** The filings you create when you file your client's nails are not healthy to breathe. If you wear a dust mask and offer one to your client, you are both protected from filing dust. Be sure to replace your mask every day because used masks lose their effectiveness very quickly. (Fig. 4.3)

5. **Wear safety glasses.** Whenever there is even the slightest chance that the chemical you are using might get into your eyes, you should wear eye protection. Always wear approved safety glasses and give your client a pair. No one ever lost business because they worked safely or showed concern for their clients' safety. (Fig. 4.4)

6. **Never wear contact lenses in the salon.** Wearing contact lenses in the salon is risky and foolish. In case of accident, it is very difficult to clean the eye if you're wearing contacts. Wearing soft contact lenses is particularly risky because vapors can collect in the soft contacts and start to bother your eyes. They can even begin to etch away the surface of the eye.

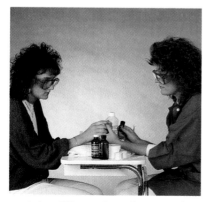

4.4 — Wear safety glasses and give your client a pair.

7. **Don't smoke in the salon.** Many of the products we use in the nail salon are highly flammable. Smoking near them could cause a fire. There should be no smoking in the area of the

salon where clients are serviced. If smoking is permitted it should be in an entirely different area. (Fig. 4.5)

8. **Never eat or drink in the salon area.** A cup of coffee is an excellent place for nail dust and powder to collect. Hot liquids like coffee and tea can absorb vapors from the air. The cup of coffee you or your client is drinking may be filled with nail chemicals. (Fig. 4.6)

9. **Store and eat your lunch in a separate area of the salon.** Where do you store your lunch before you eat it? If you put it in the same refrigerator as chemical products, your sandwich has probably absorbed a large dose of chemicals before you even get around to eating it. When you do eat lunch, you should leave the building or eat in a lunchroom that is separated from the rest of the salon by walls and a door.

10. **Always wash your hands before eating.** When someone offers you a piece of chocolate or when you dodge into the kitchen for a cookie, do you wash your hands first? If you forget to wash your hands before you grab a snack or eat lunch, you will probably end up eating the chemicals that are on your hands.

11. **Label all containers.** Every container, spray bottle, squeeze bottle, or tube in the salon must be labeled. This includes all cleaning products and any bulk purchased products in storage. Be sure the label is waterproof. If the container isn't labeled, *don't use it.* (Fig. 4.7)

12. **Store your products in a cool area.** Never store nail products in your car trunk or in an area where there is a gas heater or furnace with a pilot light. Excessive heat will ruin them, and some of them are more flammable than gasoline.

13. **Throw out the trash regularly.** The plastic trash bag that is fastened to the side of your table keeps filling your air with vapors. Each item that lives in that bag may be robbing you of the ventilation you need. Empty the trash several times a day and dispose of it properly. In most instances, you should place it in a metal container with a tight-fitting lid.

14. **Keep caps on all products.** It may seem easier to leave caps off your products, but it isn't wise. Uncapped bottles on your table are very easy to spill. Keep your product containers closed to reduce the amount of vapor that escapes into the air. Capping will also make your products last longer. Uncapped nail polish thickens, solvents evaporate, and wrap glue starts to harden. (You might find that marbles are just the right size to cover the small dishes you use for acrylic powder and liquid.)

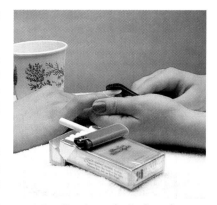
4.5 — Don't smoke in the salon; many nail products are highly flammable.

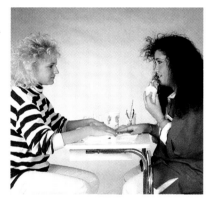
4.6 — Never eat or drink in the salon area. You may find that you're eating or drinking nail chemicals.

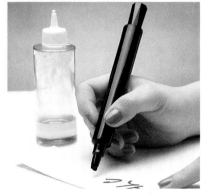
4.7 — Label all containers. If the container isn't labeled, don't use it.

38 PART I GETTING STARTED

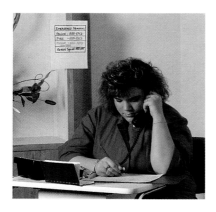

15. **Be prepared to handle accidents.** Don't wait until after an accident has happened to figure out how to handle it. Keep the MSDS for each product in a convenient place. Have the poison control number and other emergency numbers near the phone. Discuss with your coworkers what you would do in case of an accident. (Fig. 4.8)

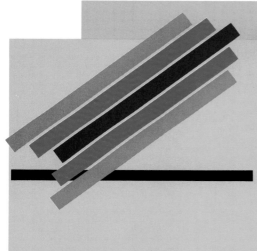

Express Yourself — Safely

Have a little fun with your safety goggles by turning them into a promotional tool for nail art. They're a great vehicle for individual expression and they're sure to attract attention. Add hand-painted designs to goggle frames or edges and change them frequently to reflect seasonal themes, color trends, and personal preference. For mini test-marketing, determine which designs generate the most interest, then offer to create those designs on your client's nails. The bottom line is that you boost your profits and create interest in nail art while promoting safety.

Review Questions

1. Name five chemicals commonly used by nail technicians in the salon.
2. What are five early warning signs of overexposure to nail chemicals.
3. What is an MSDS?
4. What is meant by the term flashpoint?
5. What are three ways that products can enter the body and cause harm?
6. What are five ways you can protect yourself and your clients when using chemicals?

PART II

THE SCIENCE OF NAIL TECHNOLOGY

- *Chapter 5 - Anatomy and Physiology*
- *Chapter 6 - The Nail and Its Disorders*
- *Chapter 7 - The Skin and Its Disorders*
- *Chapter 8 - Client Consultation*

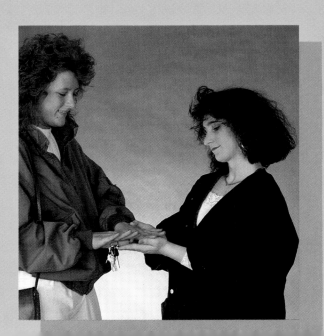

CHAPTER 5

Anatomy and Physiology

LEARNING OBJECTIVES

After you have studied this chapter, you should be able to:
1. Explain how an understanding of anatomy and physiology will help you become a better nail technician.
2. Describe the purpose of cells within the human body.
3. Describe cell metabolism and explain the difference between the two phases of metabolism.
4. Name the different types of body tissue and explain the function of each type.
5. Name the most important organs of the body and explain the function of each organ.
6. Name the systems that make up the human body and explain the function of each system.
7. List the ways in which muscles are stimulated.
8. Name the types of muscles that are affected by massage.
9. Name the divisions of the nervous system and explain the function of each division.
10. Identify the chief functions of the blood.

Introduction

Although you may have groaned when you saw a chapter on anatomy and physiology, these are important subjects in the practice of nail technology. A basic understanding of the structure of the human body and the functions it performs will give you a scientific background for many of the nail services you will learn about. This background will help you decide which service is best for a client's nail or skin condition, and how to adjust and control the service for the best results.

Very generally, anatomy is the study of the structure of the body and what it is made of—for example, bones, muscles, and skin. Physiology is the study of the small, individual structures of the body, such as hair, nails, sweat glands, and oil glands.

Although the names of bones, muscles, arteries, veins, and nerves are seldom used in the nail salon, an understanding of body structures will help make you more proficient in performing many services, such as hand and arm massage. Your study of anatomy and physiology will include cells, tissues, organs, and systems of the human body.

Cells

Cells are the basic units of all living things, including bacteria, plants, and animals. The human body is made up entirely of cells, fluids, and cellular products. As the basic functional units of all living things, the cells carry on all of our life processes. Cells also have the ability to reproduce, providing new cells that enable us to grow and that replace worn or injured tissues.

Cells are made up of **protoplasm** (**PROH**-toh-plaz-em), a colorless, jellylike substance that contains food elements such as protein, fat, carbohydrates, and mineral salts.

The **protoplasm** of the cells includes the **nucleus** (**NOO**-klee-us), cytoplasm (**SEYE**-toh-plaz-em), centrosome (**SEN**-tro-sohm), and cell membrane.

The **nucleus** is made of dense protoplasm and is found in the center of the cell within the nuclear membrane. It plays an important role in cell reproduction.

Cytoplasm is found outside of the nucleus and contains food materials necessary for the growth, reproduction, and self-repair of the cell.

The **centrosome**, a small, round body in the cytoplasm, affects the reproduction of the cell.

The **cell membrane** encloses the cytoplasm. It controls the transportation of substances in and out of the cells. (Fig. 5.1)

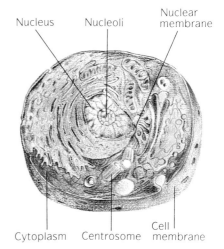

5.1 — Cells consist of protoplasm and contain essential elements.

CELL GROWTH

As long as the cell receives an adequate supply of food, oxygen, and water, eliminates waste products, and is maintained at the proper temperature, it will continue to grow and thrive. However, if these conditions do not exist and toxins (poisons) or pressure are present, then the growth and health of the cells are impaired. Most of our body cells are capable of growing and repairing themselves during their life cycle. Cells also reproduce themselves through a process of division known as mitosis. (Fig 5.2)

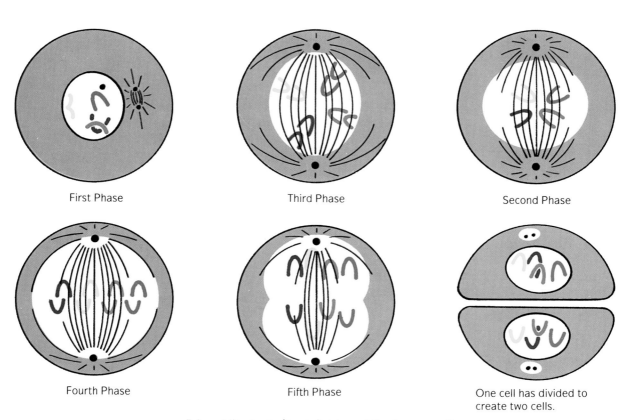

5.2 — Mitosis—indirect division of the human cell

CELL METABOLISM

Metabolism (meh-**TAB**-o-liz-em) is a complex chemical process whereby the body cells are nourished and supplied with the energy needed to carry on their many activities. There are two phases of metabolism:

1. **Anabolism** (ah-**NAB**-o-liz-em) is the process of building up larger molecules from smaller ones. During this process the body stores water, food, and oxygen for the time when these substances are needed for cell growth and repair.

2. **Catabolism** (kah-**TAB**-o-liz-em) is the breaking down of larger substances or molecules into smaller ones. This process releases energy that can be stored by special molecules for use in muscle contraction, secretion, or heat production.

Anabolism and catabolism are carried out at the same time and happen continuously. Their activities are closely regulated so that the breaking down, energy-releasing reactions are balanced with the building-up, energy-consuming reactions. Therefore, homeostasis (ho-me-oh-**STAY**-sus) (the maintenance of normal, internal stability in the body) is achieved. However, if we use less energy than we manufacture, we may notice a weight gain. The molecules of energy that are not used may turn to fat. To get rid of built-up fat, we must use more energy by exercising or take in less energy by eating less.

Tissues

Tissues are composed of groups of cells of the same kind. Each tissue has a specific function and can be recognized by its characteristic appearance. Body tissues are classified as follows:

1. **Connective tissue** serves to support, protect, and bind together tissues of the body. Bone, cartilage, ligament, tendon, fascia (which separates muscles), and fat tissue are examples of connective tissue.
2. **Muscular tissue** contracts and moves various parts of the body.
3. **Nerve tissue** carries messages to and from the brain, and controls and coordinates all body functions.
4. **Epithelial** (ep-i-**THE**-le-al) **tissue** is a protective covering on body surfaces, such as the skin, mucous membranes, linings of the ear, digestive and respiratory organs, and glands.
5. **Liquid tissue** carries food, waste products, and hormones by means of the blood and lymph.

Organs

Organs are structures designed to accomplish a specific function. The most important organs of the body are described below.

The **brain** controls the body.
The **heart** circulates the blood.
The **lungs** supply oxygen to the blood.
The **liver** removes toxic products of digestion.
The **kidneys** excrete water and other waste products.
The **stomach** and **intestines** digest food.

Systems

Systems are groups of organs that cooperate for a common purpose, namely the welfare of the entire body. The human body is made up of ten important systems.

The **integumentary** (in-**TEG**-yoo-men-ta-ree) **system,** is made up of the skin and its various accessory organs, such as the oil and sweat glands, sensory receptors, hair, and nails. This system is composed of two distinct layers, the dermis and epidermis. It functions as a protective covering and contains sensory receptors that give us our sense of touch. This system also plays an important role in regulating the temperature of the body.

The **skeletal system** is the physical foundation or framework of the body. The bones of the skeletal system serve as a means of protection, support, and locomotion (movement).

The **muscular system** covers, shapes, and supports the skeleton. Its function is to produce all the movements of the body.

The **nervous system** controls and coordinates the functions of all the other systems of the body.

The **circulatory** (**SUR**-kyoo-lah-tohr-ee) **system** supplies blood throughout the body.

The **endocrine** (**EN**-doh-krin) **system** is made up of ductless glands that secrete hormones into the bloodstream.

The **excretory** (**EK**-skre-tohr-ee) **system** eliminates waste from the body.

The **respiratory** (**RES**-pi-rah-toh-ree) **system** supplies oxygen to the body.

The **digestive system** changes food into substances that can be used by the cells of the body.

The **reproductive system** enables human beings to reproduce.

The Skeletal System

The skeletal system is the physical foundation of the body. The entire skeleton is composed of 206 bones. These bones have a variety of shapes and are connected by movable and immovable joints.

Bone, except for the tooth enamel, is the hardest tissue of the body. It is composed of connective tissues consisting of about one-third animal (organic) matter, such as cells and blood, and two-thirds mineral (inorganic) matter, mainly calcium carbonate and calcium phosphate.

The following are primary functions of the bones:
1. Give shape and support to the body.
2. Protect various internal structures and organs.

3. Serve as attachments for muscles and act as levers to produce body movements.
4. Produce various blood cells in the red bone marrow.
5. Store various minerals, such as calcium, phosphorus, magnesium, and sodium.

STRUCTURE OF BONE

Bone is white on the outside and deep red on the inside. Bone marrow is a soft, fatty, dark red substance filling the cavities of the bones. The **periosteum** (pe-ree-**OS**-tee-um) is a pink fibrous membrane that covers and protects the bone, and serves as an attachment for tendons, ligaments, blood vessels, and nerves. The blood vessels that enter the bone through the periosteum provide nutrition for the bones.

The structures attached to the bone include:

Cartilage (**CAR**-tih-ledj) is a tough elastic substance similar to bone but it has no mineral content. Cartilage cushions bones at the joints and gives shape to some external features such as the nose and ears.

Ligaments (**LIG**-e-mentz) are bands or sheets of fibrous tissue that support the bones at the joints.

Synovial (sy-**NOV**-ee-al) **fluid** is the lubrication that prevents friction at the joints where bones meet. This slippery fluid also furnishes nourishment to the cartilage.

JOINTS

The various bones of the body meet at junctions called **joints**, which can move in many ways. At **pivot** (**PIH**-vut) **joints** like the neck, one bone turns on another bone. At **hinge** (**HINJ**) **joints,** which are found in the elbow and knee, two or more bones connect like a door. At a **ball-and-socket joint** such as the hip or shoulder, one bone is rounded and fits into the socket, or hollow part, of another bone. In **gliding joints,** which are found in the ankle and wrist, two bones glide over each other.

BONES OF THE ARM AND HAND

The **scapula** (**SKAP**-yoo-lah) and the **clavicle** (**KLAV**-i-kul) form the shoulder. The clavicle is also known as the collar bone.

The **humerus** (**HYOO**-mo-rus) is the uppermost and largest bone of the arm.

The **ulna** (**UL**-nah) is the large bone on the small-finger side of the forearm.

The **radius** (**RAY**-dee-us) is the small bone in the forearm on the same side as your thumb. (Fib. 5.3)

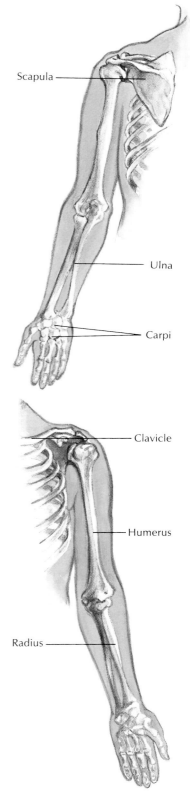

5.3 — Bones of the arm

The **carpus** (**KAHR**-pus) or wrist, is a flexible joint composed of eight small, irregular bones held together by ligaments.

The five **metacarpals** (met-a-**KAHR**-puls), the bones of the palm of the hand, are long and slender.

The **digits** or **fingers** consist of three **phalanges** (fl-**LAN**-jeez) in each finger and two in the thumb, totaling fourteen bones. (Fig. 5.4)

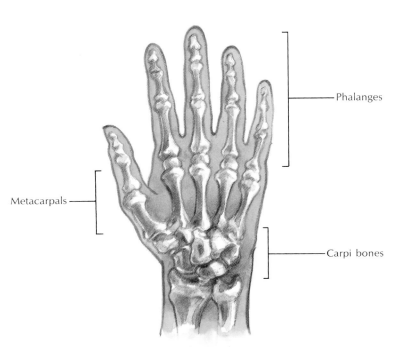

5.4 — Bones of the hand and wrist

BONES OF THE LEG AND FOOT

The **femur** (**FEE**-mur) is a heavy, long bone that forms the leg above the knee.

The **tibia** (**TIB**-ee-ah) is the larger of the two bones that form the leg below the knee.

The **fibula** (**FIB**-ya-lah) is the smaller of the two bones that form the leg below the knee.

The **patella** (pah-**TEL**-lah), also called the accessory bone, forms the knee cap. (Fig. 5.5)

The ankle is made up of seven **tarsal** (**TAR**-sul) bones. The **calcaneous** (kal-**KAY**-nee-us), or heel, is considered to be part of the ankle.

The five **metatarsals** (met-ah-**TAHR**-suls) of the foot are long and slender like the metacarpal bones of the hand.

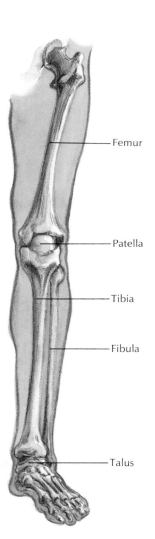

5.5 — Bones of the leg

The bones of the toes are called **phalanges** and are similar to the finger bones. There are three phalanges in each toe, except for the big toe, which has only two. (Fig 5.6)

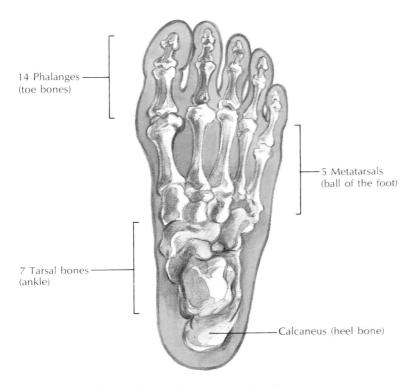

5.6 — Bones of the foot and ankle

The Muscular System

The **muscular** (**MUS**-kyoo-lahr) **system** covers, shapes, and supports the skeleton. Its function is to produce all movements of the body. **Myology** (meye-**OL**-oh-jee) is the study of the structure, functions, and diseases of the muscles.

The muscular system consists of over 500 muscles, large and small, comprising 40 to 50 percent of the weight of the human body.

Muscles are fibrous tissues that have the ability to stretch and contract according to our movements. Different types of movements —for example, stretching and bending—depend on muscles performing in specific ways.

There are three kinds of muscular tissue:

1. **Striated** (**STRY**-ate-id) muscles are voluntary muscles that you can move whenever you want. Muscles of the face, arm, and leg are striated muscles. The word striated means striped. (Fig. 5.7)

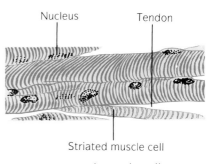

5.7 — Striated muscle cells

2. **Non-striated** muscles are involuntary. Muscles of the stomach and intestines are non-striated. These muscles function automatically. Non-striated means smooth or not striped. (Fig. 5.8)
3. **Cardiac** (**CAR**-dee-ak) muscle is heart muscle, which is not found anywhere else in the body. (Fig. 5.9)

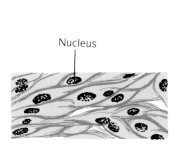

5.8 — Non-striated muscle cells

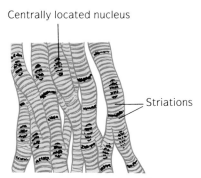

5.9 — Cardiac muscle cells

MUSCLE PARTS

There are three parts to a muscle: the origin, the insertion, and the belly. The **origin** is the part that does not move. It is attached to the skeleton, and is usually part of the skeletal muscles. The

The Magic Touch

The sense of touch is a powerful method for creating positive feelings about a particular experience. Researchers found that a simple touch on the hand gave subjects a feeling of goodwill after making store purchases and checking out library books. Subjects who were treated exactly the same, but were not touched, did not describe the experience as positive. How can you use this information to your advantage? If you include a hand massage with every manicure, your clients will feel pampered and well taken care of. Also, you can relieve retracted hand muscles for a client who types all day by simply pressing your thumb into the client's palm and holding it a few seconds. The extra attention you give will make your manicures stand out in your client's mind. Combine a silky lotion with your magic touch and your three-minute massage becomes a super business builder.

insertion is the part that moves, and the **belly** is the middle part. During a contraction, when the muscle shortens, one of the attachments usually remains fixed and the other moves. Muscles are joined together by **sinews** (**SIN**-yooz) or **tendons** (**TEN**-dunz) which look like white glistening cords.

STIMULATION OF MUSCLES

Muscle tissue can be stimulated in any of the following ways:

Massage—hand massage and electric vibrator.
Electric current—applied to the muscle area to produce visible muscle contractions.
Light rays—infrared rays and ultraviolet rays.
Heat rays—heating lamps and heating caps.
Moist heat—steamers or moderately warm steam towels.
Nerve impulses—through the nervous system.
Chemicals—certain acids and salts.

MUSCLES AFFECTED BY MASSAGE

As a nail technician, you are concerned with the voluntary muscles of the hands, arms, legs, and feet. It is essential to know where these muscles are located and what they control. Pressure in massage is usually directed from the insertion to the origin.

Muscles of the Shoulder and Upper Arm

The **deltoid** (**DEL**-toid) is a large, thick triangular muscle that covers the shoulder and lifts and turns the arm.

Biceps (**BEYE**-seps) is the muscle on the front of the upper arm that lifts the forearm, flexes the elbow and turns the palm up. It has two heads or points of attachment.

Triceps (**TREYE**-seps) are muscles that cover the entire back of the upper arm and extend the forearm forward. They have three heads or points of attachment.

Muscles of the Forearm

The **forearm** contains a series of muscles and strong tendons.

The **pronator** (**PRO**-nay-tor) turns the hands inward, so the palm faces downward.

Supinator (**SUE**-pi-nay-tor) turns the hand outward so the palm faces upward.

Flexors (**FLEKS**-ors) bend to the wrist, draw the hand upward, and close the fingers toward the forearm.

Extensor (eck-**STEN**-sur) straightens the wrist, hand, and fingers to form a straight line. (Fig. 5.10)

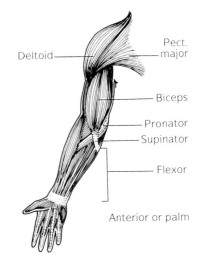
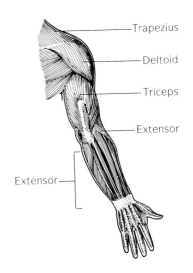

5.10 — Muscles of the arm

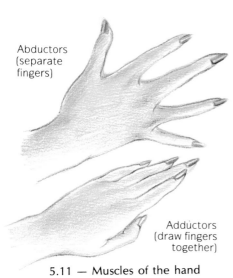

Abductors (separate fingers)

Adductors (draw fingers together)

5.11 — Muscles of the hand

Muscles of the Hand

The hand has many small muscles that overlap from joint to joint, giving flexibility and strength. When the hands are properly cared for, these muscles will remain supple and graceful. They close and open the hands and fingers.

Abductors (ab-**DUK**-tohrs) separate the fingers and **adductors** (a-**DUK**-tohrs) draw the fingers together. Both of these muscles are located at the base of the thumbs and fingers. (Fig. 5.11)

Opponent muscles are located in the palm of the hand and act to bring the thumb toward the fingers, allowing the grasping action of the hands.

Muscles of the Lower Leg and Foot

As a nail technician, you will use your knowledge of the muscles of the foot and leg during a pedicure. The muscles of the foot are small and provide proper support and cushioning for the foot and leg. (Fig. 5.12)

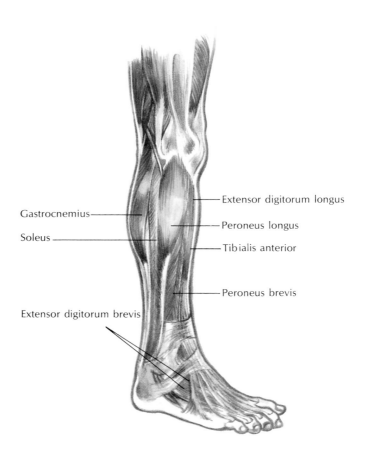

5.12 — Muscles of the lower leg and foot

The **extensor digitorum longus** (eck-**STEN**-sur dij-it-**TOHR**-um **LONG**-us) bends the foot up and extends the toes.

The **tibialis anterior** (tib-ee-**AHL**-is an-**TEHR**-ee-ohr) covers the front of the shin. It bends the foot upward and inward.

The **peroneus longus** (per-oh-**NEE**-us **LONG**-us) covers the outer side of the calf and inverts the foot and turns it outward.

The **peroneus brevis** (**BREV**-us) originates on the lower surface of the fibula. It bends the foot down and out.

The **gastrocnemius** (gas-truc-**NEEM**-e-us) is attached to the lower rear surface of the heel and pulls the foot down.

The **soleus** (**SO**-lee-us) originates at the upper portion of the fibula and bends the foot down.

The muscles of the feet include the **extensor digitorum brevis** (ek-**STEN**-sur dij-it-**TOHR**-um **BREV**-us), **abductor hallucis** (ab-**DUK**- tohr ha-**LU**-sis), **flexor digitorum brevis** (**FLEKS**-or dij-it-**tohr**-um **BREV**-us) and the **abductor**. The foot muscles move the toes and help maintain balance while walking and standing. (Fig. 5.13)

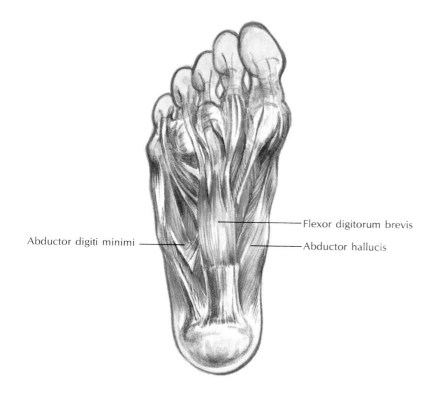

5.13 — Muscles of the foot (bottom)

The Nervous System

Neurology is the branch of medicine that deals with the nervous system and its disorders. The *nervous system* is one of the most important systems of the body. It controls and coordinates the functions of all the other systems and makes them work in harmony. Every square inch of the human body is supplied with fine fibers called **nerves**. As a nail technician, you should study the nervous system in order to understand the effect massage has on the nerves of the feet, legs, hands, arms, and the whole body.

The nervous system is composed of three divisions: the central nervous system, the peripheral system, and the autonomic nervous system.

1. The *cerebro-spinal* (ser-EE-broh SPEYE-nahl) or **central nervous system** consists of the brain and spinal cord and has the following functions.
    a) Controls consciousness and all mental activities.
    b) Controls functions of the five senses: seeing, smelling, tasting, feeling, and hearing.
    c) Controls voluntary muscle actions, such as all body movements and facial expression.
2. The *peripheral* (pe-RIF-er-al) *system* is made up of the sensory and motor nerve fibers that extend from the brain and spinal cord and are distributed to all parts of the body. Its function is to carry messages to and from the central nervous system.
3. The *autonomic* (aw-toh-NAHM-ik) *nervous system* is the portion of the nervous system that functions without conscious effort and regulates the activities of the smooth muscles, glands, blood vessels, and heart. The system has two divisions, the **sympathetic** and **parasympathetic systems,** which act in direct opposition to each other. They regulate such things as heart rate, blood pressure, breathing rate, and body temperature to aid the body in the maintenance of homeostasis, or normal internal stability. The sympathetic division is primarily activated during stressful, energy-demanding, or emergency situations; the parasympathetic division is most active in ordinary restful energy-conserving situations.

THE BRAIN AND SPINAL CORD

The brain is the largest mass of nerve tissue in the body and is contained in the cranium. The weight of the average brain is 44 to 48 ounces (1232 to 1344 g). It is considered to be the central processing unit of the body, sending and receiving digital messages. Twelve pairs of cranial nerves originate in the brain and reach various parts of the head, face, and neck.

The spinal cord is composed of masses of nerve cells, with fibers running upward and downward. It originates in the brain, extends the length of the trunk, and is enclosed and protected by the spinal column. Thirty-one pairs of spinal nerves, extending from the spinal cord, are distributed to the muscles and skin of the trunk and limbs. Some of the spinal nerves supply the internal organs controlled by the sympathetic nervous system.

NERVE CELLS AND NERVES

A *neuron* (**NOOR**-on) or *nerve cell* is the primary structural unit of the nervous system. It is composed of a cell body, **dendrites** (**DEN**-dreyets), which receive messages from other neurons, and an **axon** (**AK**-son) and **axon terminal**, which send messages to other neurons, glands, or muscles. (Fig 5.14)

Nerves are long, white cords made up of fibers that carry messages to and from various parts of the body. Nerves have their origin in the brain and spinal cord, and distribute branches to all parts of the body.

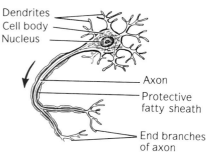

5.14 — A neuron or nerve cell

Types of Nerves

Sensory nerves, also called **afferent** (**AF**-fer-ent) **nerves,** carry impulses or messages from sense organs to the brain, where sensations of touch, cold, heat, sight, hearing, taste, smell, pain, and pressure are experienced.

Motor nerves, also called **efferent** (**EF**-fer-ent) **nerves,** carry impulses from the brain to the muscles. The transmitted impulses produce movement.

Mixed nerves contain both sensory and motor fibers and have the ability to both send and receive messages.

Sensory nerve endings, called **receptors**, are located near the surface of the skin. Impulses pass from the sensory nerves to the brain and back over the motor nerves to the muscles. A complete circuit is established and movements of the muscles result.

A *reflex* is an automatic response to a stimulus that involves the transmission of an impulse from a sensory receptor along an afferent nerve to the spinal cord, and a responsive impulse along an efferent neuron to a muscle, causing a reaction. An example of a reflex is the quick removal of the hand from a hot object. A reflex action does not have to be learned.

Nerves of the Arm and Hand

The **ulnar** (**UL**-ner) **nerve** and its branches supply the small finger side of the arm and the palm of the hand.

The **radial** (**RAY**-dee-al) **nerve** and its branches supply the thumb side of the arm and the back of the hand.

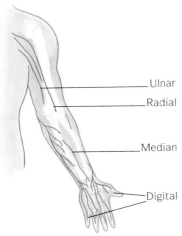

5.15 — Nerves of the arm and hand

The **median** (**MEE**-di-an) **nerve** is a smaller nerve than the ulnar and radial nerves. With its branches, it supplies the arm and hand.

The **digital** (**DIJ**-it-al) **nerve** and its branches supply all fingers of the hand. (Fig. 5.15)

Nerves of the Lower Leg and Foot

The **tibial** (**TIB**-ee-al) **nerve,** located in the thigh, passes behind the knee. It subdivides and supplies impulses to the knee, the muscles of the calf, the skin of the leg, and the sole, heel, and underside of the toes.

The **common peroneal** (per-oh-**NEE**-al) **nerve,** a division of the sciatic nerve, is located behind the knee and has two parts. The **deep peroneal nerve** passes down the back of the leg. The **superficial peroneal nerve** passes downward in front of the fibula and supplies impulses to the skin of the foot and toes.

The **saphenous** (sa-**FEEN**-us) **nerve** supplies impulses to the skin of the inner side of the leg and foot.

The **sural nerve** supplies impulses to the outer side and back of the foot and leg.

The **dorsal** (**DOOR**-sal) **nerve** supplies impulses to the top of the foot. (Fig. 5.16)

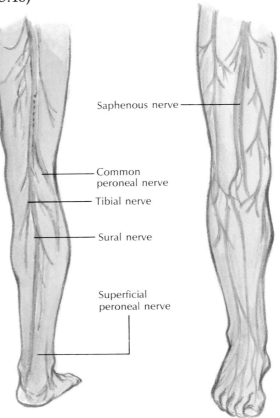

5.16 — Nerves of the lower leg and foot

The Circulatory System

The *circulatory* (**SUR**-kyoo-lah-tohr-ee), or **vascular** (**VAS**-kyoo-lahr) **system** is vital to the maintenance of good health. It controls the steady circulation of the blood through the body by means of the heart and the blood vessels (the arteries, veins, and capillaries).

The *blood-vascular system* consists of the heart and blood vessels and circulates the blood. The *lymph* (**LIMF**)-*vascular* or **lymphatic** (lim-**FAT**-ik) **system** consists of lymph glands and vessels through which a colorless fluid called lymph circulates. These two systems are intimately linked with each other. Lymph is derived from the blood and flows gradually back into the bloodstream.

THE HEART

The heart is a muscular, cone-shaped organ about the size of a closed fist. It is located in the chest cavity, and is enclosed in a membrane, the **pericardium** (per-i-**KAHR**-dee-um). It is an efficient pump that keeps the blood moving within the circulatory system. At the normal resting rate, the heart beats about 72 to 80 times a minute. The **vagus** (**VAY**-gus) (tenth cranial nerve) and nerves from the autonomic nervous system regulate the heartbeat. (Fig. 5.17)

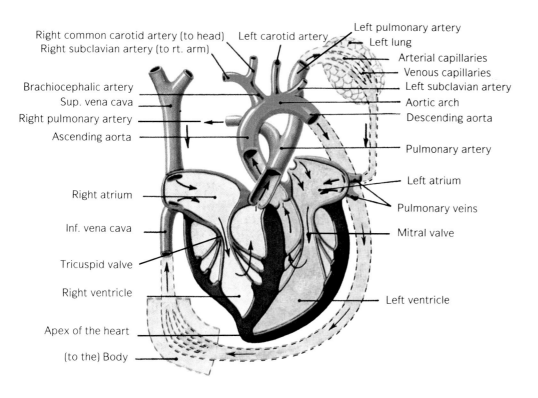

5.17 — Diagram of the heart

The interior of the heart contains four chambers and four cavities. The upper, thin-walled chambers are the **right atrium** (AY-tree-um) and **left atrium**. The lower, thick-walled chambers are the **right ventricle** (VEN-tri-kel) and **left ventricle**. **Valves** allow the blood to flow in only one direction. With each contraction and relaxation of the heart, the blood flows in, travels from the **atria** (both right atrium and left atrium) to the ventricles, and is then driven out, to be distributed all over the body. Another name for the atrium is **auricle** (OR-ik-kel).

Blood Vessels

Blood vessels, which include *arteries, capillaries,* and *veins,* are tubelike in construction. They transport blood to and from the heart and to various tissues of the body.

Arteries are thick-walled muscular and elastic tubes that carry oxygen-filled blood from the heart to the capillaries throughout the body.

Capillaries are tiny, thin-walled blood vessels that connect the smaller arteries to the veins. Through their walls, the tissues receive nourishment and eliminate waste products.

Veins carry blood that lacks oxygen from the capillaries back to the heart. They are thin-walled blood vessels that are less elastic than arteries. They contain cuplike valves to prevent backflow. Veins are located closer to the outer surface of the body than arteries are. (Fig. 5.18)

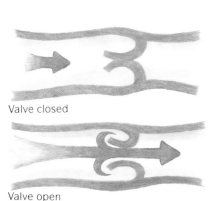

Valve closed

Valve open

5.18 — Cross-sections of a vein

THE BLOOD

Blood is a nutritive fluid that moves throughout the circulatory system. It is a red, salty fluid with a consistency similar to that of tomato juice. Blood has a normal temperature of 98.6 degrees Fahrenheit (37 degrees Celsius), and it makes up about one-twentieth of the weight of the body. Approximately 8 to 10 pints of blood fill the blood vessels of an adult. Blood is bright red in color in the arteries, except for in the pulmonary artery, and dark red in the veins (except for in the pulmonary vein). This change in color is due to the exchange of carbon dioxide for oxygen as the blood passes through the lungs and the exchange of oxygen for carbon dioxide as the blood circulates throughout the body.

Circulation of the Blood

The blood is in constant circulation from the moment it leaves the heart until it returns. There are two systems that control this circulation:

The *pulmonary* (PUL-mo-ner-ee) *circulation* is the blood circulation that goes from the heart to the lungs to be purified.

The *systemic,* or **general,** *circulation* is the blood circulation from the heart throughout the body and back again to the heart.

Composition of the Blood

The blood is composed of red and white corpuscles, platelets, and plasma. (Figs. 5.19, 5.20)

The function of **red corpuscles** (**KOR**-pus-els) (red blood cells) is to carry oxygen to the cells. **White corpuscles** (white blood cells), or **leucocytes** (**LOO**-ko-seyets), perform the function of destroying disease-causing germs.

Blood platelets (**PLAY**-tel-lets) are much smaller than the red blood cells. They play an important part in the clotting of the blood. (Fig. 5.21)

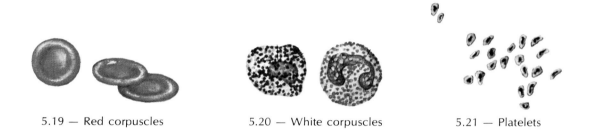

5.19 — Red corpuscles   5.20 — White corpuscles   5.21 — Platelets

Plasma is the fluid part of the blood, in which the red and white blood cells and blood platelets flow. It is straw-like in color and is about nine-tenths water. It carries food and secretions to the cells and carbon dioxide from the cells.

Chief Function of the Blood

The primary functions of the blood are described below:

1. Carries water, oxygen, food, and secretions to all cells of the body.
2. Carries away carbon dioxide and waste products to be eliminated through the lungs, skin, kidneys, and large intestine.
3. Helps to equalize the body temperature, thus protecting the body from extreme heat and cold.
4. Aids in protecting the body from harmful bacteria and infections through the action of the white blood cells.
5. Clots, thereby closing tiny, injured blood vessels and preventing the loss of blood.

Blood Supply for the Arm and Hand

The **ulnar** (**UL**-ner) and **radial** (**RAY**-dee-ul) arteries are the main blood supply for the arm and hand.

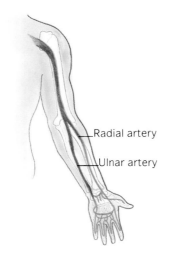

5.22 — Arteries of the hand and arm

The ulnar artery and its numerous branches supply the little-finger side of the arm and the palm of the hand. The radial artery and its branches supply the thumb side of the arm and the back of the hand.

The important veins are located almost parallel with the arteries and take the same names as the arteries. While the arteries are found deep in the tissues, the veins lie nearer to the surface of the arms, hands, legs, and feet. (Fig. 5.22)

Blood Supply to the Lower Leg and Foot

There are several major arteries that supply blood to the lower leg and foot. The **popliteal** (pop-lih-**TEE**-ul) **artery** divides into two separate arteries known as the **anterior tibial** (**TIB**-ee-al) and the **posterior tibial**. The **anterior tibial** goes to the foot and becomes the **dorsalis pedis** which supplies the foot with blood.

As in the arm and hand, the important veins of the lower leg and foot are almost parallel with the arteries and take the same names. (Fig. 5.23)

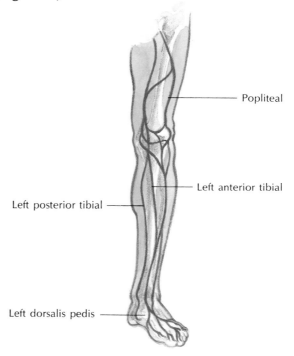

5.23 — Arteries of the lower leg and foot

The Lymph-Vascular System

The **lymph-vascular system,** also called the **lymphatic system,** acts as an aid to the blood system, and consists of lymph spaces, lymph vessels, and lymph glands.

Lymph is a colorless, watery fluid that is made from the plasma of the blood. It is created when the plasma filters through the capillary walls into the tissue spaces. The tissue fluid found in the tissue spaces bathes all cells and trades its nutritive materials to the cells in return for the waste products of metabolism. This fluid is absorbed into the lymphatics or lymph capillaries to become lymph and is then filtered and detoxified as it passes through the lymph nodes. It is eventually reintroduced into the blood circulation.

The following are the primary functions of lymph:

1. Reaches the parts of the body not reached by blood and carries on an interchange with the blood.
2. Carries nourishment from the blood to the body cells.
3. Acts as a bodily defense against invading bacteria and toxins.
4. Removes waste material from the body cells to the blood.
5. Provides a suitable fluid environment for the cells.

The Endocrine System

The *endocrine* (**EN**-doh-krin) *system* is made up of ductless glands that secrete substances into the bloodstream. A **gland** is a specialized organ that secretes substances. Glands convert certain elements from the blood into new compounds that the body needs. The **endocrine glands** secrete **hormones,** chemicals that affect metabolism and other body processes, directly into the bloodstream. The endocrine system works with the nervous system to regulate and integrate the various organs and systems of the body.

The Excretory System

The *excretory* (**EK**-skr-tohr-ee) *system,* including the kidneys, liver, skin, intestines, and lungs, purifies the body by eliminating waste matter.

Each of the following plays a part in the excretory system:

1. **Kidneys** excrete urine.
2. The **liver** discharges bile.
3. The **skin** eliminates perspiration.
4. The **large intestine** evacuates decomposed and undigested food.
5. The **lungs** exhale carbon dioxide.

Metabolism of the cells of the body forms various toxic substances which, if retained, might poison the body.

The Respiratory System

The *respiratory system* is situated within the chest cavity, which is protected on both sides by the ribs. The **diaphragm** is a muscular partition that controls breathing, and separates the chest from the **abdominal** region.

The **lungs** are spongy tissues composed of microscopic cells that take in air. These tiny air cells are enclosed in a skin-like tissue. Behind this, the fine capillaries of the vascular system are found.

When we breathe, an exchange of gases takes place. When we **inhale,** oxygen is absorbed into the blood. Carbon dioxide is expelled when we **exhale.** Oxygen is more essential than either food or water. Although a person may live more than 60 days without food, and a few days without water, if deprived of oxygen, he or she will die in a few minutes.

Breathing through your nose is healthier than breathing through your mouth because the air is warmed by the surface capillaries and the bacteria in the air are caught by the hairs that line the mucous membranes of the nasal passages.

Your rate of breathing depends on your level of activity. Muscular activities and energy expenditures increase the body's demands for oxygen. As a result, the rate of breathing is increased. You require about three times more oxygen when walking than when standing.

The Digestive System

Digestion is the process of converting food into a form that can be used by the body. The **digestive system** changes food into **soluble** form, suitable for use by the cells of the body. Digestion begins in the mouth and is completed in the small intestine. From the mouth, the food passes down the **pharynx** (**FAR**-ingks) and the **esophagus** (i-**SOF**-a-gus), or food pipe, and into the stomach. The food is completely digested in the stomach and small intestine and is assimilated or absorbed into the bloodstream. The large intestine (colon) stores the refuse for elimination through the rectum. The complete digestive process of food takes about 9 hours.

Enzymes, which are present in the digestive secretions, are responsible for the chemical changes in food. **Digestive enzymes** are chemicals that change certain kinds of food into a form capable of being used by the body. Intense emotions, excitement, and fatigue seriously disturb digestion. On the other hand, happiness and relaxation promote good digestion.

Review Questions

1. How can an understanding of anatomy and physiology help you become a better nail technician?
2. What is the purpose of cells within the human body?
3. What is cell metabolism?
4. Name the five types of body tissue and explain the function of each.
5. What are the five most important organs of the body? Explain the function of each.
6. List the ten systems that make up the human body. What is the function of each system?
7. What are four ways in which muscles are stimulated?
8. What are four types of muscles that are affected by massage?
9. What are the three divisions of the nervous system? What is the function of each division?
10. What are the chief functions of the blood?

CHAPTER 6

The Nail and Its Disorders

LEARNING OBJECTIVES

After you have studied this chapter, you should be able to:
1. *Identify the parts of the nail.*
2. *Define the term nail disorder.*
3. *Cite the golden rule for dealing with nail disorders.*
4. *Identify the nail disorders that can be serviced by a nail technician.*
5. *Identify the nail disorders that cannot be serviced by a nail technician.*

Introduction

To give your clients professional and responsible service and care, you need to learn about the structure and function of the nails. You also must be able to know when it is safe to work on a client and when they need to see a dermatologist, a medical doctor who is a skin specialist.

Nails are an interesting and surprising part of the human body. They are small mirrors of the general health of the body. Healthy nails are smooth, shiny, and translucent pink. Systemic problems in the body can show in the nails as nail disorders or poor nail growth. The technical term for nail is *onyx* (**ON**-iks). Nails are a part of the skin and are made of the same protein, **keratin** (**KER**-a-tin), as skin and hair. Nails are composed of the hardest keratin. Hair is made of a hard keratin, but not as hard as the keratin in nails, and skin is made of soft keratin. The purpose of nails is to protect the ends of fingers and toes and to help the fingers grasp small objects. Adult fingernails grow at an average rate of 1/8 inch a month; toenails grow more slowly.

Nails replace themselves every five to six months and grow more quickly in summer than in the winter. The nail grows fastest on the middle finger and slowest on the thumb.

Parts of the Nail

The entire nail structure consists of parts of the actual nail and structures of skin beneath and surrounding the nail.

PARTS OF THE NAIL

The actual nail consists of the nail body, nail root, and free edge. The *nail body* or *plate* is the main part or plate of nail that is attached to the skin at the tip of the finger. Although the nail plate appears to be one piece, it is actually constructed of layers. (Fig. 6.1)

The *nail root* is where the nail growth begins. It is embedded underneath the skin at the base of the nail.

The *free edge* is the end of the nail that extends beyond the fingertip.

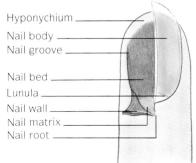

6.1 — Diagram of the nail

STRUCTURES BENEATH THE NAIL

The structures beneath the nail include the nail bed, matrix, and lunula. The *nail bed* is the portion of skin beneath the nail body that the nail plate rests upon. The nail bed is supplied with blood vessels that provide the nourishment necessary for nail growth. The nail bed also contains nerves. (Fig. 6.2)

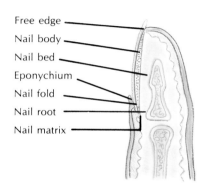

6.2 — Cross section of the nail

The *matrix* (**MAY**-triks) contains nerves together with lymph and blood vessels that produce nail cells and control the rate of growth of the nail. It is located under the nail root. The matrix is a very sensitive part of the nail and if injured will produce nails with irregular growth and disorders. Be careful not to apply excessive pressure to this area during a manicure.

The *lunula* is the light-colored half-moon shape at the base of the nail. This is where the matrix connects with the nail bed.

SKIN SURROUNDING THE NAIL

The skin surrounding the nail includes the cuticle, nail fold, nail grooves, nail wall, eponychium, paronychium, and hyponychium.

The *cuticle* (**KYOO**-ti-kel) is the overlapping skin around the nail. A normal cuticle should be loose and pliable.

The *nail fold* or *mantle* (**MAN**-tel) is the deep fold of skin at the base of the nail where the nail root is imbedded.

The *nail grooves* are slits or tracks in the nail bed at the sides of the nail on which the nail grows.

The *nail wall* is the skin on the sides of the nail above the grooves.

The *eponychium* (ep-o-**NIK**-ee-um) is the thin line of skin at the base of the nail that extends from the nail wall to the nail plate.

The *paronychium* (par-oh-**NIK**-ee-um) is the part of the skin that surrounds the entire nail area.

The *hyponychium* (heye-poh-**NIK**-ee-um) is the part of the skin under the free edge of the nail.

Nail Disorders

A *nail disorder* is a condition caused by injury to the nail or disease or imbalance in the body. Most, if not all, of your clients have had some type of common nail disorder and may have one when they are scheduled for a manicure. As a nail technician, you learn to recognize the symptoms of nail disorders so you can make a responsible decision about whether you should perform a service on your client.

You may be able to help your clients with nail disorders in one of two ways. You can tell clients that they may have a disorder and refer them to a physician. In other cases you can cosmetically improve a nail disorder and improve the overall beauty of your clients' nails.

It is your responsibility to know when it is safe to work on your clients' nails. You must learn to recognize the symptoms of nail disorders that cannot be worked on. In addition, you must know when to treat nails with extra care and when you can perform a service to cosmetically improve a disorder. Use the "golden rule" to make a responsible decision about the health of your clients' nails.

"**The golden rule**" is that, if the nail or skin to be worked on is infected, inflamed, broken, or swollen, a nail technician should not service the client. Instead refer the client to a doctor. An *inflammation* (in-flam-**MAY**-shun) is red and sore. An *infection* (in-**FEK**-shun) will have evidence of pus. Inflammation and infection are not the same thing, although they often occur at the same time. *Broken* skin or nail tissue is a cut or tear that exposes deeper layers of these structures. *Raised* or *swollen* skin will appear fatter than normal skin and rise above the normal level.

The lists below contain the names of nail disorders and a short description of each one. The first list contains the names of nail disorders that nail technicians can work on if there is no evidence of infection, inflammation, broken tissue, or swelling. The list also suggests services you might perform. The second list contains descriptions of nail disorders that are too serious for a nail technician to work on and that must be referred to a physician.

NAIL DISORDERS THAT CAN BE SERVICED BY A NAIL TECHNICIAN

Bruised nails is a condition in which a clot of blood forms under the nail plate. The clot is caused by injury to the nail bed. It can vary in color from maroon to black. In some cases, a bruised nail will fall off during the healing process. Applying artificial nail services to a bruised nail is not recommended. (Fig. 6.3)

Discolored nails is a condition in which the nails turn a variety of colors including yellow, blue, blue-grey, green, red, and purple. Discoloration can be caused by poor blood circulation, a heart condition, or topical or oral medications. It may also indicate the presence of a systemic disorder. Artificial tips or wraps or an application of colored nail polish can hide this condition.

Eggshell nails are thin, white, and curved over the free edge. The condition is caused by improper diet, internal disease, medication, or nervous disorders. Be very careful when manicuring these nails because they are fragile and can break easily. Use the fine side of an emery board to file gently and do not use pressure with a metal pusher at the base of the nail. (Figs. 6.4, 6.5)

Furrows, also known as corrugations, are long ridges that run either lengthwise or across the nail. Some lengthwise ridges are normal in adult nails, and they increase with age. Lengthwise ridges can also be caused by conditions such as psoriasis, poor circulation, and frostbite. Ridges that run across the nail can be caused by conditions such as high fever, pregnancy, measles in childhood, and a zinc deficiency in the body. If ridges are not deep and the nail is not broken, you can correct the appearance of this disorder.

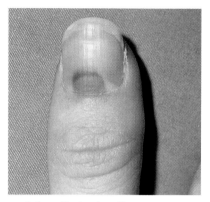

6.3 — Bruised nail

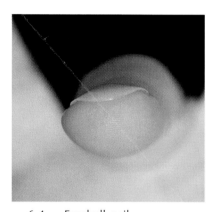

6.4 — Eggshell nail

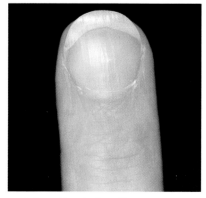

6.5 — Eggshell nail

66 PART II THE SCIENCE OF NAIL TECHNOLOGY

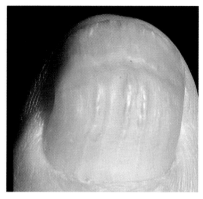

6.6 — Furrows or corrugations

Carefully buff the nails with pumice powder to remove or shorten the ridges. The remaining ridges can be filled with ridge filler and covered with colored polish to give a smooth, healthy look to the nail. (Fig. 6.6)

Hangnails, also known as agnails, is a common condition in which the cuticle around the nail splits. Hangnails are caused by dry cuticles or cuticles that have been cut too close to the nail. This disorder can be improved by softening the cuticles with oil and trimming the cuticles with nippers. Though this is a simple and common disorder, hangnails can become infected if not serviced properly. (Fig. 6.7)

Leuconychia (loo-ko-**NIK**-ee-ah) is a condition in which white spots appear on the nails. It is caused by air bubbles, a bruise, or other injury to the nail. Leuconychia cannot be corrected, but it will grow out. (Fig. 6.8)

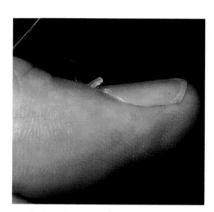

6.7 — Hangnail

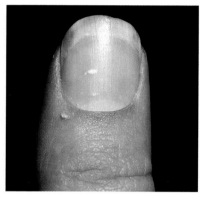

6.8 — Leuconychia

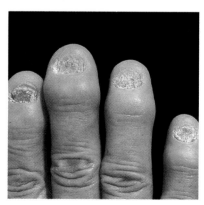

6.9 — Onychatrophia or atrophy of the nail

Nevus (**NEE**-vus) is a brown or black stain on the nail caused by a pigmented mole that occurs in the nail. Nail polish or an artificial nail service can hide this disorder.

Onychatrophia (on-i-kah-**TROH**-fee-ah), also known as atrophy describes the wasting away of the nail. The nail loses it shine, shrinks, and falls off. Onychatrophia can be caused by injury to the nail matrix or by internal disease. Handle this condition with extreme care. File the nail with the fine side of the emery board and do not use a metal pusher or strong soaps or washing powders. If the condition is caused by internal disease and the disease is cured, new nails may grow back. (Fig. 6.9)

Onychauxis (on-i-**KIK**-sis) or *hypertrophy* (hy-**PER**-troh-fee) shows the opposite symptoms of onychatrophia. Onychauxis is the overgrowth of nails. Nails with this disorder are abnormally thick. The condition is usually caused by internal imbalance, local infection, or heredity. File the nail smooth and buff it with pumice powder. (Figs. 6.10, 6.11)

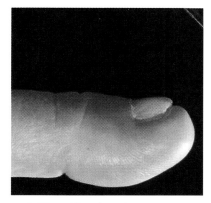

6.10 — Onychauxis

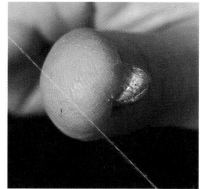

6.11 — Onychauxis (end view)

Onychocryptosis (on-i-koh-krip-**TOH**-sis) or *ingrown nails* is a familiar condition of the fingers and toes in which the nail grows into the sides of the tissue around the nail. Improper filing of the nail and poor-fitting shoes are causes of this disorder. If the tissue around the nail is not infected or if the nail is not too deeply imbedded in the flesh, you can trim the corner of the nail in a curved shape to relieve the pressure on the nail groove. If the nail has grown very deeply into the groove, refer the client to a physician. (Fig. 6.12)

Onychophagy (on-i-**KOH**-fa-jee) is the medical term for nails that have been bitten enough to become deformed. This condition can be improved greatly by professional manicuring techniques. Give frequent manicures, using the techniques described in the manicuring chapters of this book. As those chapters suggest, any of the artificial tips and wraps can hide and beautify deformed nails. (Fig. 6.13)

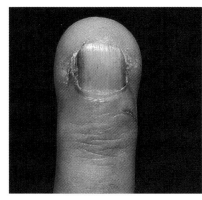

6.12 — Onychocryptosis or ingrown nail

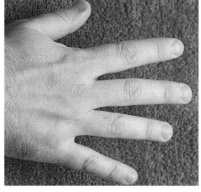

6.13 — Bitten nails or onychophagy

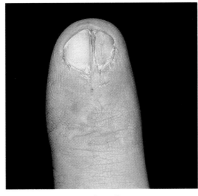

6.14 — Onychorrhexis

Onychorrhexis (on-i-kohr-**REK**-sis) refers to split or brittle nails that also have a series of lengthwise ridges. It can be caused by injury to the fingers, excessive use of cuticle solvents, nail polish removers, and careless, rough filing. Nail services can be performed only if the nail is not split below the free edge. This condition may be corrected by softening the nails with a reconditioning treatment and discontinuing the use of harsh soaps, polish removers, or improper filing. (Fig. 6.14)

Pterygium (te-**RIJ**-ee-um) describes the common condition of the forward growth of the cuticle on the nail. The cuticle sticks to the nail and, if not treated, will grow over the nail to the free edge.

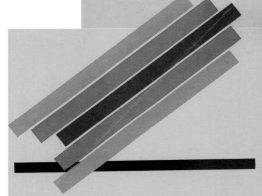

Hard-Bitten Advice

Nail biting bites into your business. To help clients overcome this compulsion, try these five salon-tested techniques from nail technicians who found them to be successful:

- Recommend a weekly manicure and promote your treatments for nail biters. Once clients see the difference, nail pride grows and, along with it, a determination to control the habit.
- Apply tips or wraps. They feel surprisingly different in the mouth and the shock discourages nail biters.
- Suggest that your client try acupuncture. It's been known to be very successful in controlling compulsive behaviors such as smoking, overeating, and nail biting.
- Apply similar nail art to all ten nails. With the first bite, the continuity of the art is destroyed, which acts as a negative reinforcement and discourages nail biting.
- Develop a six-week program and have clients pay for all six visits up front to make a commitment. At each visit, treat the cuticles and nails, discuss ways to avoid situations that bring on biting, and then send clients home with nail-biting liquids and bitter-tasting herbs to apply to nails.

This condition can easily be treated by a reconditioning hot oil manicure, which will soften the cuticle so it can be pushed back by the metal pusher and then removed. (Fig. 6.15)

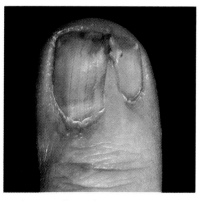

6.15 — Pterygium

NAIL DISORDERS THAT CANNOT BE SERVICED BY A NAIL TECHNICIAN

Mold is a fungus infection of the nail that is usually caused when moisture seeps between an artificial nail and the free edge of the nail. Mold starts with a yellow-green color and darkens to black if not treated by a doctor. A client with mold must be referred to a doctor. (Fig. 6.16)

Onychia (on-**NIK**-ee-ah) is an inflammation somewhere in the nail. The tissue at the base of the nail may be red and swollen and pus may form. It is often caused by improperly sanitized manicuring implements. (Fig. 6.17)

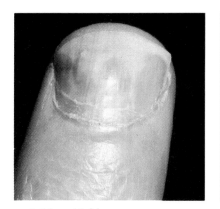

6.16 — Mold

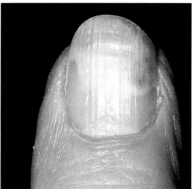

6.17 — Onychia

Onychogryphosis (on-i-koh-greye-**FOH**-sis) is a conditon in which the nail curvature is increased and enlarged. The nail becomes thicker and curves, sometimes extending over the tip of the finger or toe. This condition results in inflammation and pain if the nail grows into the skin. The cause of this disorder is unknown.

Onychomycosis (oni-koh-meye-**KOH**-sis), *tinea unguim* (**TIN**-ee-ah **Un**-gwee-um), of the nails, is an infectious disease caused by a fungus (vegetable parasite). A common form is whitish patches

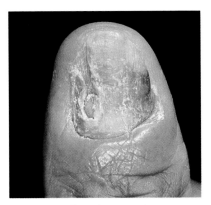

6.18 — Onychomycosis

that can be scraped off the surface. A second form is long, yellowish streaks within the nail substance. The disease invades the free edge and spreads toward the root. The infected portion is thick and discolored. In a third form, the deeper layers of the nail are invaded, causing the superficial layers to appear irregularly thin. These infected layers peel off and expose the diseased parts of the nail bed. (Fig. 6.18)

Onycholysis (on-i-**KOL**-i-sis) is a condition in which the nail loosens from the nail bed, beginning usually at the free edge and continuing to the lunula, but does not come off. It is caused by an internal disorder, trauma, infection, or certain drug treatments. It can occur on the nails of the hands or feet. (Figs. 6.19, 6.20)

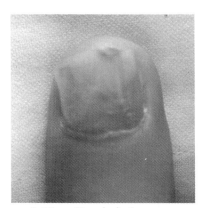

6.19 — Onycholysis (caused by trauma)

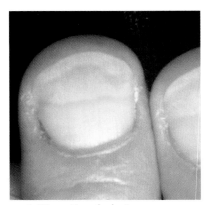

6.20 — Onycholysis

Onychoptosis (on-i-kop-**TOH**-sis) is a condition in which part or all of the nail sheds periodically and falls off the finger. It is a condition that can affect one or more nails. It can occur during or after certain diseases of the body, such as syphilis, as a result of fever and system upsets, as a reaction to prescription drugs, or as a result of trauma.

Paronychia (par-oh-**NIK**-ee-ah) is a bacterial inflammation of the tissue around the nail. The symptoms are redness, swelling, and tenderness of the tissue surrounding the nail.

Paronychia can occur at the base of the nail, around the entire nail plate, or on the fingertip. Paronychia around the entire nail is sometimes referred to as runaround. Chronic paronychia occurs continually over a long period of time and causes damage to the nail plate. Paronychia can be caused by the use of unsanitary implements or by aggressive pushing or cutting of the cuticle. (Figs. 6.21, 6.22, 6.23)

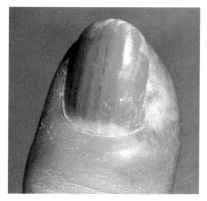

6.21 — Paronychia

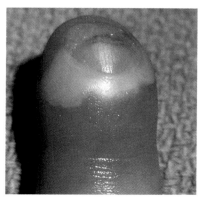

6.22 — Paronychia (runaround)

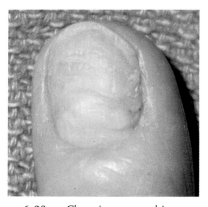

6.23 — Chronic paronychia

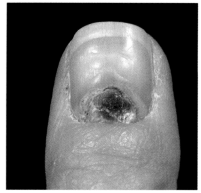

6.24 — Pyrogenic granuloma

Pyrogenic granuloma is a severe inflammation of the nail in which a lump of red tissue grows up from the nail bed to the nail plate. (Fig. 6.24)

Review Questions

1. What are the three parts that make up the nail?
2. Define nail disorder.
3. What is the golden rule for dealing with nail disorders?
4. List five nail disorders that can be serviced by a nail technician.
5. List five nail disorders that cannot be serviced by a nail technician.

CHAPTER 7

The Skin and Its Disorders

LEARNING OBJECTIVES

After you have studied this chapter, you should be able to:
1. Describe the characteristics of healthy skin.
2. List the functions of the skin.
3. Describe the epidermis and dermis.
4. Explain how the skin is nourished.
5. Describe the function of sweat glands.
6. Define lesion.
7. Describe the characteristics of eczema and psoriasis.

Introduction

As a nail technician you must have a basic understanding of the skin and its disorders in order to serve your clients responsibly and professionally. You will have the opportunity to improve the appearance of the skin on the hands and feet and therefore to enhance your client's appearance. The finished nails will look their best when set off by beautiful, healthy skin. In addition, it is your responsibility to know when you cannot work on a client or must not use certain products on your client due to a skin condition. Knowledge of the skin will help you avoid the spread of infectious disease and aggravation of skin conditions or sensitivities. Before you can judge whether a particular service or product is appropriate for your client's skin, you must have a general understanding of what the skin is and how it functions. Because the nails are an appendage of the skin, problems with the skin can cause nail problems.

Healthy Skin

To be a nail technician, you must learn about ***dermatology*** (der-mah-**TOL**-o-jee), the study of healthy skin and skin disorders. Healthy skin is slightly moist and acid, soft and flexible. Unless the skin is aged, healthy skin has ***elasticity*** that allows it to regain its shape immediately after being pulled away from the bone. Healthy skin is free of blemishes and disease and its texture is smooth and fine-grained. The skin on the human body varies in thickness. It is thinnest on the eyelids and thickest on the palms of the hands and soles of the feet.

FUNCTION OF THE SKIN

The skin performs eight jobs for the body. They include protection, the prevention of fluid loss, response to external stimuli, heat regulation, secretion, excretion, absorption, and respiration.

1. **Protection.** The skin covers every part of the body and protects it from injury and invasion by bacteria.

2. **Prevention of fluid loss.** The skin seals blood and other bodily fluids inside the body.

3. **Response to *external stimuli*.** The skin contains nerve endings that respond to stimuli from outside the body, such as heat,

cold, touch, pressure, and pain. This sensitivity helps the body find the most comfortable environment.

4. **Heat regulation.** The skin keeps the body's internal temperature at 98.6 degrees Fahrenheit (37 degrees Celsius). When the temperature outside the body changes, the blood and sweat glands of the skin heat or cool the body to maintain its temperature.

5. **Secretion.** The oil (sebaceous) glands secrete **sebum**, a fatty, oily substance that maintains the skin's moisture level by slowing the evaporation of moisture from the skin and preventing excess water from penetrating the skin.

6. **Excretion.** The sweat (sudoriferous) glands excrete salt and other waste chemicals from the body through the pores of the skin (perspiration).

7. **Absorption.** The skin absorbs small amounts of chemicals, drugs, and cosmetics through the pores.

8. **Respiration.** The skin breathes through the pores. Oxygen is absorbed and carbon dioxide is discharged.

STRUCTURE OF THE SKIN

The skin has two layers or parts. The outer layer is called the epidermis; the deep layer under the epidermis is called the dermis. (Figs. 7.1, 7.2)

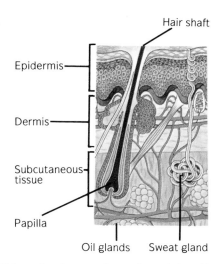

7.1 — A microscopic section of the skin

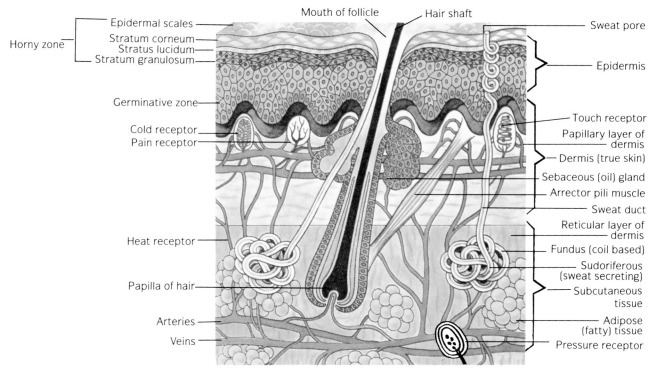

7.2 — Diagram of the skin

Epidermis

The *epidermis* (ep-i-**DUR**-mis), also called the *cuticle* or *scarf skin*, is the outermost protective covering of the skin. It contains no blood vessels, but contains many small nerve endings. The epidermis is made of the following four layers:

The *stratum corneum* (**STRAT**-um **KOHR**-nee-um), also called the **horny layer**, which consists of tightly packed, scalelike cells that are continually shed and replaced. These cells form keratin, the substance that makes up skin, nails, and hair. The keratin also acts as a waterproof coating for the skin.

The *stratum lucidum* (**STRAT**-um **LOO**-si-dum) is a small layer of clear cells that light can pass through.

The *stratum granulosum* (**STRAT**-um gran-yoo-**LOH**-sum) consists of cells that look like granules. These cells change into keratin near the surface of the skin.

The *stratum germinativum* (**STRAT**-um jur-mi-nah-**TIV**-um), formerly known as the *stratum mucosum* (**STRAT**-um myoo-**KOH**-sum), can also be referred to as the basal of Malpighian layer. This layer is composed of several layers of differently shaped cells. The deepest layer is responsible for supplying new cells to make up for the ones that are continually worn away. It also contains a dark skin pigment, called *melanin* (**MEL**-a-nin), which determines skin color and protects the sensitive cells below from the destructive effects of excessive ultraviolet rays from the sun or an ultraviolet lamp.

The Dermis

The **dermis** is the deep layer of the skin and is also called the "true skin," **derma, corium,** or **cutis.** Blood vessels and lymph vessels, nerves, sweat glands, and oil glands are contained in this layer in an elastic network made up of collagen. The dermis contains three separate layers.

The *papillary* (**PA**-pil-ah-ry) *layer* lies directly under the epidermis and contains the *papillae* (pa-**PIL**-e), little cone-like projections that extend upward into the epidermis. Some of the papillae contain looped capillaries, and small blood vessels; others contain nerve endings. This layer also contains some of the melanin pigment.

The *reticular* (re-**TIK**-u-lar) *layer* contains fat cells, blood and lymph vessels, sweat and oil glands, and hair follicles.

The *subcutaneous* (sub-kyoo-**TAY**-nee-us) *tissue* is made up of fatty tissue known as *adipose* (**AD**-i-pohs). This tissue gives smoothness and shape to the body, contains a store of fat to be burned for energy, and acts as a protective cushion for the outer skin. It varies in thickness according to the age, sex, and general health of the individual.

NOURISHMENT OF THE SKIN

The skin is nourished by blood and lymph. See Chapter 5 for more information about blood and lymph. One-half to two-thirds of the total blood supply of the body is distributed to the skin. The blood and lymph supply essential nourishment for growth and repair of skin, hair, and nails. The subcutaneous layer of the skin contains arteries and lymphatic vessels that send small branches to provide nourishment to hair papillae, hair follicles, and skin glands. The skin also contains numerous capillaries.

NERVES OF THE SKIN

A *nerve* is made of cordlike fibers and sends messages from the body organs to the central nervous system which consists of the brain and the spinal cord. The skin contains the surface endings of many nerve fibers.

These nerve ending are called *tactile corpuscles* (**TAK**-til **KOR**-puh-sils) and they perform the following functions:

Motor nerves move the blood vessels and the *arrectores pili* (a-**REK**-tohr **PIGH**-ligh) muscles that are attached to the hair follicles. These muscles can cause goose bumps.

Sensory nerves, which are found in the papillary layer of the dermis, give the skin a sense of touch They allow you to react to heat, cold, touch, pressure, and pain. Sensory nerve endings are most abundant in the fingertips. Complex sensations, such as vibrations, seem to depend on the sensitivity of a combination of these nerve endings. (Fig. 7.3)

Secretory (se-**KREET**-e-ree) *nerves* are the nerves of the sweat and oil glands.

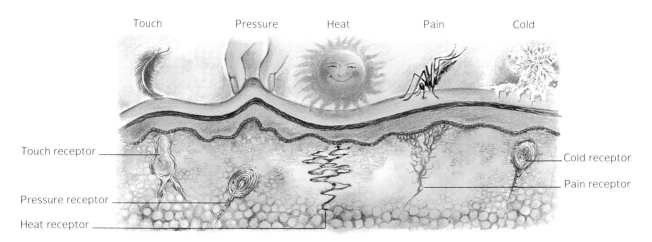

7.3 — Sensory nerves of the skin

GLANDS OF THE SKIN

The skin contains two types of duct glands that extract materials from the blood and turn them into different substances. These new substances are secreted for use by the body or excreted from the body.

The *sudoriferous* (su-dohr-**IF**-er-us) *glands*, or sweat glands, regulate body temperature and eliminate waste products through perspiration. Though the nervous system controls the excretion of sweat, activity is greatly increased by heat, exercise, emotions, and certain drugs. One to two pints of liquids containing salts are normally eliminated daily through the sweat pores in the skin. (Fig. 7.4)

Sweat glands consist of a coiled base, called a *fundus* (**FUN**-dus) and a tubelike duct that ends at the skin surface to form a *sweat pore*. A sweat pore is a small opening in the skin surface from which the sweat gland eliminates waste. Most parts of the body have sweat glands. The palms of the hands, soles of the feet, forehead, and armpits have the greatest number of sweat glands.

The *sebaceous* (si-**BAY**-shus) or *oil glands* secrete an oily substance, called sebum, as you learned earlier in this chapter.

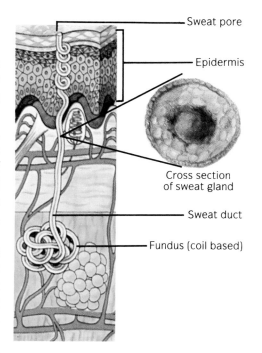

7.4 — Sudoriferous or sweat glands

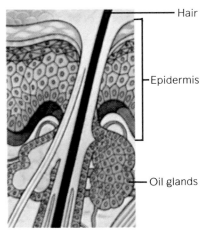

7.5 — Sebaceous or oil glands

Sebum lubricates the skin and softens the hair. All parts of the body except the palms of the hands and soles of the feet have oil glands. The oil glands consist of little sacs with ducts that open into the hair follicles. When the oil gland produces sebum in the sac, it flows through the oil duct into the hair follicle. If the sebum hardens and the duct becomes clogged, a **blackhead** forms. Cleansing skin regularly will prevent the oil ducts from clogging. (Fig. 7.5)

ELASTICITY OF THE SKIN

The *elastic tissue* in the papillary layer of the dermis gives the skin its ability to return to its original shape after it has been stretched. As a person ages, the papillary tissue begins to lose its elastic nature. The skin begins to sag or wrinkle because it no longer can return to its original shape.

Skin Disorders

As a nail technician, you need to learn about skin disorders so you can decide when it is safe and appropriate to work on a client. Your goal is to prevent the spread of an infectious disease and to avoid worsening a condition your client already has. You will observe the skin of a client during the consultation and use your special knowledge to make an informed decision about servicing your client. While only a medical doctor is qualified to make a diagnosis, you should learn to recognize the symptoms that indicate that a disorder is present. It is difficult to recognize some skin disorders in practice, so you must use the following ''golden rule'' when making your decision.

The golden rule of skin disorders is that if the area of skin to be worked on is infected, inflamed, broken, or raised, a nail technician should not service the client. The client should be referred to a dermatologist. **Inflamed skin** is red, sore, and swollen. Inflamed skin is *not* the same as infected skin. **Infected skin** will have evidence of pus. **Broken skin** occurs when the epidermis is cut or torn, exposing the deeper layers of skin. **Raised skin** is a symptom of a variety of skin conditions, some of which are lesions, and will be described below. If the skin is raised at all, do not work on it; refer your client to a physician.

LESIONS OF THE SKIN

A *lesion* (**LEE**-zhun) is a structural change in tissue caused by injury and disease. While studying the different skin lesions, remember that you will always use your "golden rule" to decide whether or not it is safe to work on your client. (Fig. 7.6)

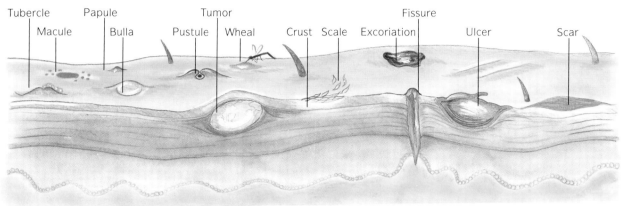

7.6 — Lesions of the skin

A *bulla* (**BYOO**-lah) is a blister containing watery fluid.

A *crust* is an accumulation of serum and pus mixed with epidermal flakes. An example of crust is a scab on a sore.

A *cyst* (**SIST**) is a semisolid or fluid lump above and below the skin surface.

Excoriation (ed-skohr-i-**AY**-shun) is a sore or abrasion caused by scratching or scraping.

A *fissure* (**FISH**-ur) is a crack in the skin that penetrates the dermis. Chapped hands or lips are an example.

A *macule* (**MAK**-ul) is a small, discolored spot or patch on the surface of the skin. Some macules are safe and some are not.

A *papule* (**PAP**-yool) is a small pimple that does not contain fluid, but can develop pus.

A *pustule* (**PUS**-chool) is a lump on the skin with an inflamed base and a head containing pus.

Scales are produced during the shedding of the epidermis. Severe dandruff is an example of scales.

A *scar* is a light-colored, slightly raised mark on the skin formed after an injury or lesion of the skin has healed.

A *stain* is an abnormal discoloration that remains after moles, freckles, or liver spots disappear, or after certain diseases.

A *tubercle* (**TOO**-ber-kyool) is a solid lump larger than a papule. It varies in size from a pea to a hickory nut.

A *tumor* is an abnormal cell mass that varies in size, shape, and color. *Nodules* are small tumors.

An *ulcer* (**UL**-ser) is an open lesion on the skin or mucous membrane of the body. Ulcers are accompanied by pus and loss of skin depth.

A *vesicle* (**VES**-i-kell) is a blister containing clear fluid. Poison ivy is an example of a condition that produces vesicles.

Wheals (**HWEELS**) or *hives* are swollen, itchy bumps on the skin that last for several hours. They are often caused by insect bites or by allergic reactions.

INFLAMMATIONS OF THE SKIN

There are several types of *inflammations* of the skin, also known as dermatitis. If inflammation, infection, or raised or broken skin is present, do not work on the inflamed area. Be very cautious when working on a client who suffers from these disorders because the skin is sensitive and the condition can be aggravated by the use of chemicals.

Eczema (**EK**-se-mah) is a chronic, long-lasting disorder of unknown cause. It is characterized by itching, burning, and the formation of scales and oozing blisters.

Psoriasis (so-**REYE**-a-sis) is a chronic inflammation with round, dry patches covered with coarse silvery scales. It is usually found on the scalp, elbows, knees, chest, and lower back; rarely on the face.

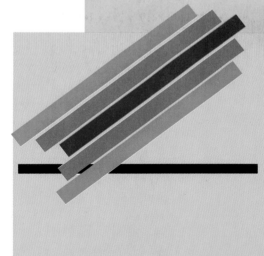

The Dip That Refreshes

To keep your client's skin looking and feeling healthy, offer a paraffin treatment. This service requires a minimal investment (wax and a heater) and provides maximum return. After the client's nail polish has been removed, massage the hands or feet with a rich emollient and dip each hand or foot into heated paraffin wax. Repeated dipping, with a few seconds between each immersion in the wax, causes the wax to build up slowly in layers and seals the lotion. After five to seven dips, wrap the hands or feet in plastic bags, slip them into insulated mits, and ask your client to relax. After ten minutes, peel the wax off, much like a glove or a bootie. Your client's hands or feet will look healthy and feel soft and you'll be able to charge $10 or more for this refreshing ten-minute service.

CHAPTER 7 THE SKIN AND ITS DISORDERS 81

INFECTIONS OF THE SKIN

You cannot perform nail services on a customer who has either a fungus infection or a viral infection of the skin. Clients with either type of infection should be referred to a physician.

Athlete's foot, also known as tinea pedis (**TIN**-ee-ah **PEH**-dus) or ringworm of the foot, is a fungus infection of the foot. The symptoms are small, pink spots or blisters and itching around the toes and on the sole of one or both feet. In extreme cases the nail can become infected. Athlete's foot is highly contagious and should not be touched by a nail technician. (Fig. 7.7)

Herpes simplex is a skin infection common in dental staff and others involved with care of the mouth. It may start as painful paronychia (see Chapter 6). This is a serious viral infection that may occur periodically. (Fig. 7.8)

Ringworm (tinea) of the hand is a highly contagious disease caused by a fungus. The principal symptoms are red lesions occurring in patches or rings over the hands. Itching may be slight or severe. (Fig. 7.9)

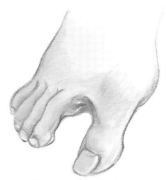
7.7 — Athlete's foot

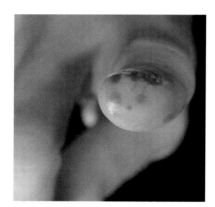
7.8 — Herpes simplex

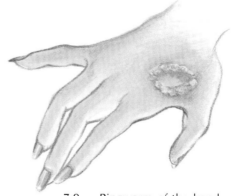
7.9 — Ringworm of the hand

Pigmentation of the Skin

The color of the skin is determined in part by the blood supply to the skin, but mostly by melanin, or coloring matter. Abnormal pigmentary conditions may be caused by internal or external factors. Certain medications are also known to cause pigmentary irregularities. Clients with these irregularities can receive nail services.

Albinism (**AL**-bi-niz-em) is a congenital absence of melanin pigment in the body, including the skin, hair, and eyes. The hair is silky white. The skin is pinkish white and does not tan. The eyes are pink and the skin ages early. Albinism is a form of *leucoderma* (loo-ko-**DER**-ma), a general term for the abnormal lack of pigmentation.

Chloasma (kloh-**AZ**-mah) are brown spots on the skin, especially the face and hands. Chloasma are also called "liver spots" or "moth patches."

Lentigines (len-ti-**JEE**-neez), or *freckles*, are small brown or yellow spots.

A *birthmark* or *nevus* (**NEE**-vus) is a malformation of the skin due to abnormal pigmentation or dilated capillaries. The condition may be inherited.

A *tan* is the darkening of the skin caused by exposure to the ultraviolet rays of the sun.

Vitiligo (vit-l-**EYE**-go) is an acquired form of leucoderma that affects the skin or hair. People with vitiligo must be protected from the sun.

Hypertrophies (New Growths) of the Skin

A *keratoma*, or callus, is an acquired superficial, round and thickened patch of epidermis due to pressure or friction on the hands and feet. If the thickening grows inward it is called a corn.

A *mole* is a small, brown spot on the skin. Moles are believed to be inherited. They range in color from pale tan to brown or bluish black. Some moles are small and flat and look like freckles. Others are raised and darker than freckles in color. Moles often have hairs growing out of them. **Do not touch or remove hair from moles.**

Melanotic sarcoma is a fatal skin cancer that begins with the growth of a mole. A physician should be consulted immediately if there is any change in a mole.

Review Questions

1. What are the characteristics of healthy skin?
2. What are five functions of the skin?
3. Describe the epidermis and dermis.
4. How is the skin nourished?
5. What are the functions of sweat glands?
6. Name five types of lesions.
7. What are the characteristics of eczema and psoriasis?

CHAPTER
8

Client Consultation

LEARNING OBJECTIVES

After you have studied this chapter, you should be able to:
1. *Explain the purpose of a client consultation.*
2. *Describe the appearance of healthy nails.*
3. *Explain why knowing a client's lifestyle is helpful in making decisions about products and services.*
4. *Determine when it is necessary to refer a client to a physician.*
5. *Describe the information that should be gathered on the client health/record card.*

Introduction

Before you perform a service on a client, you should take time to talk with that client and complete a client health/record card and a client service record. During this conversation, called the **client consultation**, you will discuss the client's general health, the health of his or her nails and skin, the client's lifestyle and needs, and the nail services that you can perform. You will use your knowledge of skin, nails, and each type of nail service to help your client select the most appropriate service. If the client has a nail or skin disorder that prevents you from performing a service, you should refer that client to a physician and offer to perform a service as soon as the disorder has been treated. A good client consultation is the difference between being a professional and just "doing nails."

Determining the Condition of Nails and Skin

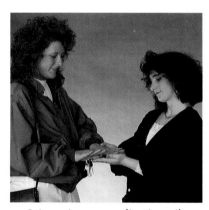

8.1 — Are your client's nails and skin healthy?

Are your client's nails and skin healthy? Look at the nails and skin of the hands or feet (depending on the service). Examine them for disorders. Generally, if there is no inflammation, infection, swelling, or broken skin it is okay to work on that client. It may be necessary to refer a client to a physician if you find a problem. It is important to handle this situation very delicately. (Fig 8.1)

If you need to refer a client to a physician, you must act responsibly and tactfully. Explain to your client that you think there may be a problem and to be safe you will not perform a service until the client has visited a doctor. Never attempt to diagnose the problem because you could cause unnecessary stress for your client. While it may be difficult to turn a client away, you must do so. Performing a service on an infected nail could cause great pain to your client, for which you would be blamed. In addition, your client will be impressed with your professionalism and concern for health and safety.

Does your client have allergies? You should always try to avoid using products that can cause an allergic reaction. If your client does have a reaction to a product, be sure to make a note on his or her client health/record card that includes both the product and the type of reaction.

Determining Your Client's Needs

What nail service does the client want? If your client asks for a specific nail service, discuss the procedure used to create that service, the benefits, and proper maintenance. Make sure that your client's expectations are realistic. Keep this desired service in mind as you discuss the client's lifestyle. You may know of a nail service that is better suited to the client's needs.

What kind of lifestyle does the client have? What kind of job does your client have? What hobbies? Are your client's hands often in water? Does your client walk a lot? By learning the answers to these types of questions, you will be able to decide such things as the best length for your client's nails or how much callus to remove from the feet. Is the client a gardener, model, guitar player, or runner? A gardener might need short nails because it would be difficult to remove dirt from under a long nail. Dirt that cannot be removed can lead to infection or a painful break. A guitar player may need short nails on the left hand and want longer nails on the right hand. He or she also needs calluses on the fingertips of the left hand. A model needs beautiful nails and skin. (Fig 8.2) A runner may have calluses on the feet that protect the feet during running. You must always consider your client's personality styles and activities when choosing a nail service. (Fig 8.3) In each of these cases the wrong service could make a client unhappy and even cause pain. You're the professional; it's your job to make the client happy. If your client gets a service and is not happy with it, he or she may not return. If you offer a different service than was originally requested and explain why you feel that service is better suited for the client, you will have that client for life.

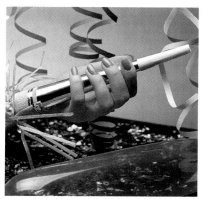
8.2 — A model needs beautiful nails.

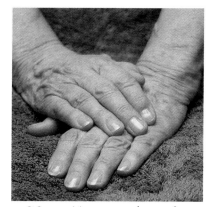
8.3 — Many people prefer natural looking nails.

Meeting Your Client's Needs

What is the client's final decision about nail services? After talking with your client about his or her needs, expectations, and nail health you will either confirm the client's service choice or recommend another service. At this time, explain why this service is best for the client, what you will do during the procedure, and what results the client can expect. For example, you would not want your client to believe that nail wraps stayed on forever and needed no maintenance. The client would be very disappointed, despite having a very professional service, when the wrap began to grow out. This is the appropriate time to explain any safety precautions you will take during the procedure. For example, if you are going

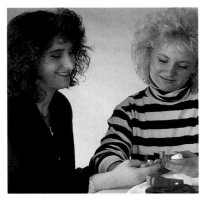

8.4 — Explain why you think a particular service is best for your client.

to apply acrylic nails, you should explain why you will wear safety goggles while applying primer. It is also a good idea to offer your client the same protection. (Fig 8.4)

After you have completed this process with your client you will start the procedure. You and your client can be sure that it is the appropriate service. Time and money are being spent wisely. The nail service will not conflict with the client's lifestyle and should meet all expectations; your client will also know that you are concerned about health and safety. Your client will leave your salon as a satisfied client and will also return to you again and again as a steady client!

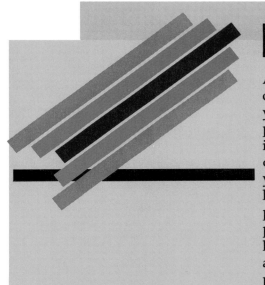

Know When to Say No

A good consultation sometimes includes referral to other professionals when an existing problem is one you can't solve. Never perform a manicure or pedicure if the nail or skin to be worked on is infected, inflamed, broken, or swollen. Keep a list of dermatologists in your area, and tactfully suggest that your client visit one that's conveniently located. Be honest about your inability to solve your client's particular problem and emphasize that once the problem clears up, you can help him or her maintain healthy hands and feet through regular manicures and pedicures. Nail technicians who follow this procedure say that clients are so appreciative that they usually return to the salon and become loyal customers.

Completing the Client Health/Record Card

Client health/record cards will vary from one salon to another. These cards should be kept in a convenient location where they can provide ready reference for every nail technician in the salon. If the salon is computerized, health/record information can be kept on computer and accessed by making a few simple keystrokes.

CLIENT HEALTH/RECORD CARD

Name: _____

Home address: _____ Work address: _____

Home telephone: _____ Work telephone: _____

Best hours for appointment are: _____

CLIENT PROFILE

1. What type of work do you do?
   _____

2. Do you have any hobbies that require you to work with your hands?
   _____

3. Do you participate in sports activities? If so, what type?
   _____

4. Do you wear rubber gloves when doing housework?
   _____

5. How much time do you spend each week caring for your own nails?
   _____

6. How frequently do you have professional nail services?
   _____

MEDICAL RECORD

Do you have:	NO	YES
Arthritis	____	____
Cancer	____	____
Diabetes	____	____
Heart problems	____	____
High blood pressure	____	____

If you answered yes to any of the above questions, what kind, if any, of medication do you take?
_____

Have you ever had a stroke? If so, how long ago?
_____

Are there any other medical conditions or medications that we should be aware of?
_____
_____

CLIENT SERVICE RECORD

Name: _____

Home address: _____ Work address: _____

Best hours for appointment are: _____

DATE	SERVICE PERFORMED	OBSERVATIONS	PRICE

DATE	RETAIL PRODUCTS SOLD	PRICE

What future nail services were discussed?
_____
_____
_____

Client health/record cards usually include three valuable types of information:

General information asks for the client's name, address, telephone number, and preferred appointment hours.

The **client profile** asks for information about the type of work and leisure activities the client participates in.

The **medical record** asks for information about the client's general health. This information will help you determine whether it is safe to perform nail services or hand and foot massage on the client.

Maintaining the Client Service Record

Each time a client receives a service in the salon, an entry should be made in the client service record. This record is usually kept on an index card and includes information about services performed, retail products sold, and future nail services discussed.

The client service record is a valuable record for the salon to maintain in case a client comes in for a nail service when his or her usual nail technician is not available.

Both the client health/record card and the client service record are client consultation tools that tell your clients that you are professional. As a professional you care about health, safety, and the quality of the services your clients receive.

Review Questions

1. What is the purpose of a client consultation.
2. What are the characteristics of healthy nails?
3. How would your services differ for a runner or a guitar player?
4. Under what circumstances would you refer a client to a physician?
5. What are the three types of information on the client health/record card?

PART III

BASIC PROCEDURES

- *Chapter 9 - Manicuring*
- *Chapter 10 - Pedicuring*

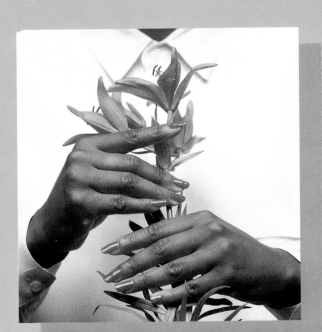

CHAPTER 9

Manicuring

LEARNING OBJECTIVES

After you have studied this chapter, you should be able to:
1. *Identify the equipment, implements, materials, and cosmetics needed for a manicure and explain what they are used for.*
2. *Describe the basic table set-up.*
3. *Describe the four basic nail shapes.*
4. *List the steps in the pre-service procedure for a water manicure.*
5. *Demonstrate the proper procedure and precautions for a water manicure.*
6. *List the steps in the post-service procedure for a water manicure.*
7. *Describe the five types of polish application.*
8. *Demonstrate the proper procedure and precautions for the reconditioning hot oil manicure.*
9. *Describe the steps in a man's manicure.*
10. *Demonstrate your ability to perform hand and arm massage properly.*

Introduction

The information and procedures you learn in this chapter will give you the basic skills to be a professional nail technician. When you master these skills and use them with your clients, you will gain the confidence and efficiency needed to develop a loyal clientele. The first step of this learning process is to become acquainted with the tools of your trade. The four types of nail technology tools are:

1. Equipment
2. Implements
3. Materials
4. Nail Cosmetics

Nail Technology Supplies

EQUIPMENT

Permanent items used in nail technology are called equipment. They can be used for all your services and do not have to be replaced until they wear out.

Manicure table with adjustable lamp. Most standard manicuring tables will include a drawer (for storing sanitized implements and cosmetics) and will have an attached, adjustable lamp. The lamp should have a 40 watt bulb. The heat from a higher wattage bulb will interfere with manicuring and sculptured nail procedures. A lower wattage bulb will not be able to warm a client's nails in a room that is highly air conditioned. The warmth from the bulb will help you maintain product consistency.

Client's chair and nail technician's chair or stool.

Fingerbowl. A plastic, china, or glass bowl that can be specially shaped for soaking the client's fingers in warm water and antibacterial soap. (Fig. 9.1)

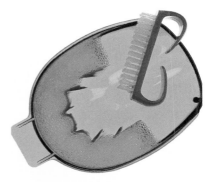

9.1 — Fingerbowl filled with warm water and antibacterial soap and nail brush

Wet sanitizer. A receptacle large enough to hold the disinfectant solution in which objects to be sanitized are immersed. A cover is provided with most wet sanitizers to prevent contamination of the solution when it is not in use. (Fig. 9.2)

Client's cushion. The cushion can be 8 by 12 inches and especially made for manicuring; a towel that is folded to cushion size can also be used. The cushion or folded towel should be covered with a clean, sanitized towel before each appointment.

Sanitized cotton container. This container will hold clean, absorbent cotton.

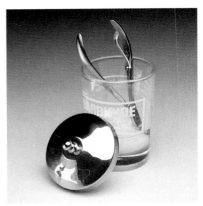

9.2 — Wet sanitizer

Supply tray. The tray holds cosmetics such as polishes, polish removers, and creams.

Electric nail dryer. A nail dryer is an optional item used to shorten the length of time necessary for the client's nails to dry.

IMPLEMENTS

Implements are tools that must be sanitized or disposed of after use with each client. They are small enough to be sanitized in a wet sanitizer.

Orangewood stick. Use the orangewood stick to loosen cuticle around the base of a nail or to clean under the free edge. Hold the stick as you would a pencil. When you use it to apply cosmetics, wrap a small piece of cotton around the end. (Fig. 9.3)

Steel Pusher. The steel pusher, also called a cuticle pusher, is used to push back excess cuticle growth. Hold the steel pusher the way you hold a pencil. The spoon end is used to loosen and push back cuticle. If you have rough or sharp edges on your pusher, use an emery board to dull them. This prevents digging into the nail plate. (Fig. 9.4)

Metal nail file. A metal nail file is used to shape the free edge of hard or sculptured nails. Most professional nail technicians use 7"–8" nail files because some states do not allow shorter files to be used. Since a nail file is metal and reusable, it must be sanitized after each use. When using a nail file, hold it with your thumb on one side of the handle and four fingers on the other side. (Fig. 9.5)

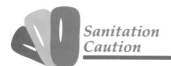

Sanitation Caution

If you drop an orangewood stick on the floor, it must be discarded. It is a disposable implement that cannot be sanitized or reused.

Sanitation Caution

The cotton on your orangewood stick needs to be changed after each use.

STATE REGULATION ALERT

Some states do not permit nail technicians to use metal nail files. Be guided by your instructor.

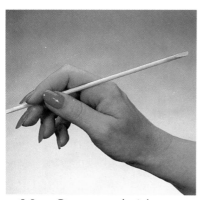

9.3 — Orangewood stick

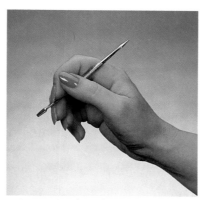

9.4 — Steel pusher

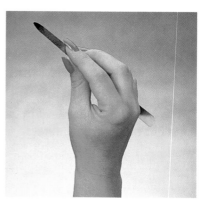

9.5 — Metal nail file

Emery board. Many nail technicians prefer an emery board to a nail file. It is also a good choice for filing soft or fragile nails, because it is not as coarse as a nail file. An emery board has two sides, a coarse-grained side and a fine-grained side. The coarse side is used to shape the free edge of the nail, and the fine side is used to bevel the nail or smooth the free edge. Hold the emery board the way you hold a nail file, with the wider end in your hand so you can file with the narrow end. To bevel, hold the emery board at a 45 degree angle and file, using light pressure, on the top or underside of the nail. Most professional nail technicians use 7"–8" emery boards because some states do not allow the use of smaller ones. The emery board cannot be sanitized, so you must either give it to your client or break it in half and discard it after use. It is *not* a good idea to save an emery board in a plastic bag for each client. Bacteria can grow on the unsanitized implement before your client's next appointment. (Fig. 9.6)

Cuticle nipper. A cuticle nipper is used to trim away excess cuticle at the base of the nail. To use the nippers, hold them in the palm of your hand with the blades facing the cuticle. Place your thumb on one handle and three fingers on the other handle, with your index finger on the screw to help guide the blade around cuticle. (Fig. 9.7)

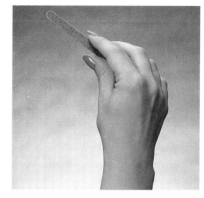

9.6 — Emery board

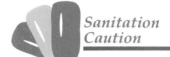

Sanitation Caution

If you drop an emery board on the floor during a procedure, it must be discarded. This is a disposable item and cannot be reused or sanitized.

STATE REGULATION ALERT

Some states do not permit nail technicians to clip cuticles. Be guided by your instructor.

Tweezers. Tweezers are used to lift small bits of cuticle from the nail.

Nail Brush. A nail brush is used to clean fingernails and remove bits of cuticle with warm soapy water. Hold the nail brush with the bristles turned down and away from you. Place your thumb on the handle side of the brush that is facing you and your fingers on the other side.

Chamois buffer. The chamois (**SHAM**-ee) buffer is used to add shine to the nail and to smooth out corrugations or wavy ridges on nails. There are two types of chamois buffer. The first has an open handle; the second has a closed handle on the top. To use the open-handled buffer, place your fingers around the handle with your thumb on the side of the handle to help guide it. To use the closed-handled type, rest your thumb along the edge of the buffer

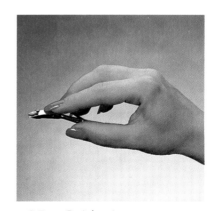

9.7 — Cuticle nippers

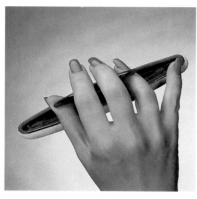

9.8 — Holding a nail buffer

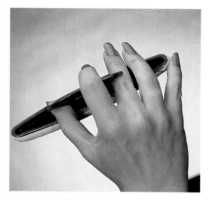

9.9 — Alternative way to hold a nail buffer

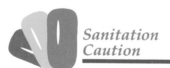

Sanitation Caution

Your chamois buffer must be designed so the chamois can be changed for each client. Be sure to discard the used chamois after each use.

to guide and support your use of this implement. Another way to hold a closed-handled chamois buffer is to place the middle and ring fingers through the closed-handled buffer if it has an open slot. Be guided by your instructor on how to hold the chamois buffer. (Figs. 9.8, 9.9)

STATE REGULATION ALERT

Some states do not permit the use of a chamois buffer. Be guided by your instructor.

Fingernail clippers. Fingernail clippers are used to shorten nails. If your client's nails are very long, clipping cuts filing time.

Sanitation for Implements

It is a good idea to have two complete sets of metal implements, so you will always have a completely sanitized set for each client, with no waiting between appointments. If you have only one set of implements, remember that it takes twenty minutes to sanitize implements after each use. A few sanitation hints are given below. For a complete discussion of sanitation, see pages 23–41.

- Wash all implements thoroughly with soap and warm water and rinse off all traces of soap with plain water. Dry thoroughly with a sanitized towel.
- Metal implements should be immersed in a wet sanitizer with cotton at the bottom and filled with an approved disinfectant. The required sanitation time is usually 20 minutes. Dry the implements with a sanitized towel when you remove them from the wet sanitizer.
- Follow your state regulations for storage of sanitized manicuring implements. The regulations will tell you to store them in sealed containers, sealed plastic bags, or in a cabinet sanitizer until they are ready for use.

STATE REGULATION ALERT

In some states, it is a violation of sanitary codes to have metal implements on your table when not in use. Be guided by your instructor about proper storage.

MATERIALS

Materials are supplies that are used during a manicure and need to be replaced for each client.

Disposable towels or terry cloth towels. A fresh, sanitized terry towel is used to cover the client's cushion before each manicure. Another fresh towel should be used to dry the client's hands after soaking in the fingerbowl. Other terry or lint-free disposable towels are used to wipe spills that may occur around the fingerbowl.

Cotton or cotton balls. Cotton is used to remove polish, wrap the end of the orangewood stick, and apply nail cosmetics. Some nail technicians prefer to use small fiber-free squares to remove polish because they don't leave cotton fibers on the nails that might interfere with polish application.

Plastic spatula. The spatula is used to remove nail cosmetics from their containers. Always use your plastic spatula, not your fingers, to remove cosmetics. A closed container of nail cosmetics is a perfect place for bacteria from your fingers to grow.

Plastic bags. Tape or clip a bag to the side of the manicuring table to hold the used materials you discard during a service. Line all trash cans with plastic bags. Be sure to have a generous supply of bags so you can change them regularly during the day.

Alcohol. Alcohol is used as a disinfectant for your manicure table and implements. Consult your state cosmetology department for information about the required strength.

Powdered alum or styptic powder. Powdered alum, or styptic (**STIP**-tik) powder, is used to contract the skin to stop minor bleeding that may occur during a manicure. To use, blot cut with powdered alum on a cotton-tipped orangewood stick.

STATE REGULATION ALERT

Styptic pencils are not permitted for use in most states because they are unsanitary.

NAIL COSMETICS

As a professional nail technician, you need to know how to use each nail cosmetic and what ingredients it contains. You need to know how to apply each cosmetic and when to avoid using a product because of a client's allergies or sensitivities. In this section you will learn what some of the basic nail cosmetics are, what each product does, and the basic ingredients each contains.

Antibacterial soap. This soap is mixed with warm water and used in the fingerbowl. It contains a soap or detergent and an antibacterial agent to sanitize the client's hands. It comes in four forms: flaked, beaded, cake, and liquid.

Polish remover. Polish remover is used to dissolve and remove nail polish. It usually contains organic solvents and acetone. Sometimes, oil is added to offset the drying effect of the acetone. Use non-acetone polish remover for clients who have artificial nails, because acetone will weaken or dissolve tips, wrap glues, and sculptured nail compound.

Cuticle cream. Cuticle cream is used to lubricate and soften dry cuticles and brittle nails. It contains fats and waxes, such as lanolin, cocoa butter, petroleum, and beeswax.

Cuticle oil. Cuticle oil keeps the cuticle soft and helps to prevent hangnails or rough cuticles. It gives an added touch to the finish of a manicure. Cuticle oil contains ingredients such as vegetable oil, vitamin E, mineral oil, jojoba, and palm nut oil. Suggest that your clients use it at bedtime to keep their cuticles soft.

Cuticle solvent or cuticle remover. Cuticle solvent makes cuticles easier to remove and minimizes clipping. It contains 2–5 percent sodium or potassium hydroxide plus glycerin.

Nail bleach. Apply nail bleach to nail plate and under free edge to remove yellow stains. It contains hydrogen peroxide. If nail bleach cannot be purchased, use 20 volume (6 percent) hydrogen peroxide.

> **STOP** *Safety Caution*
>
> Care must be taken not to get nail bleach on cuticles or skin because it can cause irritation.

Nail whitener. Nail whiteners are applied under the free edge of a nail to make the nail appear white. They contain zinc oxide or titanium dioxide. Nail whiteners are available in a paste, cream, coated string, and pencil form.

STATE REGULATION ALERT

Nail white pencils are not permitted in most states because they are unsanitary.

Dry nail polish. Dry nail polish, or **pumice** (**PUM**-is) powder is used with the chamois buffer to add shine to the nail. Some clients prefer it to liquid clear polish. Dry nail polish contains mild **abrasives** (ah-**BRAY**-sihvs), which are used for smoothing or sanding, such as tin oxide, talc, silica, and kaolin. Dry nail polish is available in powder and cream form.

Colored polish, liquid enamel, or lacquer (**LAK**-er). Colored polish is used to add color and gloss to the nail. It is usually applied in two coats. Colored polish contains a solution of nitrocellulose in a volatile solvent, such as amyl acetate and evaporates easily. Manufacturers add castor oil to prevent the polish from drying too rapidly.

Base coat. The base coat is colorless and is applied to the natural nail before the application of colored polish. It prevents red or dark polish from yellowing or staining the nail plate. Base coat is the first polish you apply in the polish procedure, unless you are using a nail strengthener. It contains more resin than colored polish to maintain a tacky surface so the colored polish will adhere better. It contains ethyl acetate, a solvent, isopropyl alcohol, butyl acetate, nitrocellulose, resin, and sometimes formaldehyde.

Nail strengthener/hardener. Nail strengthener is applied to the natural nail before the base coat. It prevents splitting and peeling of the nail. There are three types of nail strengthener:

Protein hardener is a combination of clear polish and protein, such as collagen.

Nylon fiber is a combination of clear polish with nylon fibers. It is applied first vertically and then horizontally on the nail plate. It can be hard to cover because the fibers on the nail are visible.

Formaldehyde strengthener contains 5 percent formaldehyde.

Top coat or sealer. The top coat, a colorless polish, is applied over colored polish to prevent chipping and add a shine to the finished nail. It contains nitrocellulose, toluene (**TOL**-yoo-een), a solvent, isopropyl alcohol, and polyester resins.

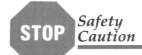

Safety Caution

All nail polishes are flammable.

Liquid nail dry. Liquid "nail dry" is used to prevent smudging of the polish. It promotes rapid drying so that the polish is not tacky and prevents the polish from dulling. It has an alcohol base and is available in brush-on or spray.

Hand cream and hand lotion. Hand lotion and hand cream add a finishing touch to a manicure. Since they soften and smooth the hands, they make the finished manicure as beautiful as possible. Hand cream helps the skin retain moisture, so hands are not dry, cracked, and wrinkled. Hand cream is thicker than hand lotion and is made of emollients and humectants, such as glycerin, cocoa butter, lecithin, and gums. Hand lotion has a thinner consistency than hand cream because it contains more oil. In addition to oil, hand lotion contains stearic acid, water, mucilage of quince seed as a healing agent, lanolin, glycerin, and gum. Hand cream or hand lotion can be used as oil in a reconditioning hot oil manicure.

Nail conditioner contains moisturizers, and should be applied at night before bedtime to help prevent brittle nails and dry cuticles.

Procedure for Basic Table Set-Up

It is important that your manicure table is sanitary and properly equipped with implements, materials, and cosmetics. Anything you need during a service should be at your fingertips. Having an orderly table will give you and your client confidence during the manicure. The actual placement of supplies on the manicuring table is a suggestion. Since regulations regarding table set-up vary from state to state, be guided by your instructor. To set up your table, use the following procedure.

1. Wipe manicure table with approved disinfectant.

2. Wrap your client's cushion in a clean, sanitized towel, either terry cloth or disposable. Put it in the middle of the table so the cushion is towards the client and the end of towel is towards you.

3. Put cotton in the bottom of the wet sanitizer. Then fill the wet sanitizer with alcohol 20 minutes before your first manicure of the day. Put all metal implements into the wet sanitizer. Place the wet sanitizer to your right if you are right-handed, or to your left if you are left-handed.

4. Put the cosmetics (except polish) on the right side of the table behind your wet sanitizer (if left-handed, place on left).

5. Put emery boards and chamois buffer on the table to your right (if left-handed, to the left).

6. Put fingerbowl and brush in the middle or to the left, towards the client. The fingerbowl or hot oil heater should not be moved from side to side of the manicure table. It should stay where you put it for the duration of your manicure. If you're doing a reconditioning hot oil manicure, replace fingerbowl and brush with electric hot oil heater.

7. Tape or clip a plastic bag to right side of table (if left-handed, tape to left side). This is used for depositing used materials during your manicure.

8. Put polishes to the left (if left-handed, place on right).

9. Your drawer can be used to keep the following items: extra cotton or cotton balls in their original container or in a fresh plastic bag; pumice stone or powder; extra chamois for buffer; instant nail dry or other supplies. Be sure to wipe drawer with

alcohol before putting supplies in it. Never place used materials in your drawer. Only completely sanitized implements (sealed in air-tight containers) and extra materials or cosmetics should be placed in this drawer. Always keep it clean and sanitary. (Fig. 9.10)

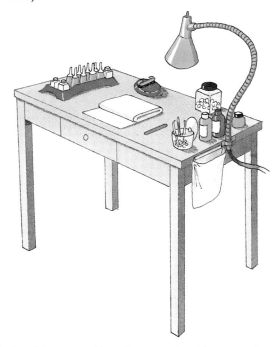

9.10 — Basic table set-up. Your instructor's table set-up is equally correct.

Choosing a Nail Shape

After the client consultation, you will discuss what shape and color nails your client wants. Keep the following considerations in mind: the shape of the hands, length of fingers, shape of the cuticles, and the type of work clients do. The following are four shapes from which to choose. (Fig. 9.11)

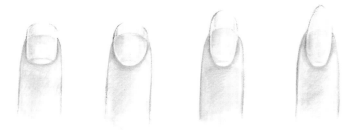

9.11 — The four basic nail shapes: rectangular, round, oval, and pointed.

- The *rectangular or square nail* should extend only slightly past the tip of the finger with the free edge rounded off. This shape is sturdy because the full width of the nail remains at the free edge. Clients who work with their hands—on a typewriter, computer, or assembly line—will need shorter, square nails.
- The *round nail* should be slightly tapered and extend just a bit past the tip of the finger. Round nails are the most common choice for male clients because of their natural shape.
- The *oval nail* is an attractive nail shape for most women's hands. It is a square nail with slightly rounded corners. Professional clients who have their hands on display (professional business people, teachers, or salespeople, for example) may want longer oval nails.
- The *pointed nail* is suited to thin hands with narrow nail beds. The nail is tapered somewhat longer than usual to enhance the slender appearance of the hand; however, these nails are weak and break easily.

Water Manicure

As a professional nail technician, you will follow a three-part procedure for all services you perform. First, in the Pre-Service, you will sanitize, greet your client, and do a client consultation. Next you will do the steps in the actual Procedure. Then, in the Post-Service, you will schedule another appointment for your client, sell the retail products you have suggested during the service, and sanitize.

WATER MANICURE PRE-SERVICE

1. **Do your Pre-Service Sanitation Procedure.** (This procedure is described on pages 29–30.)
2. **Set up your standard manicuring table.**
3. **Greet client.** (Fig. 9.12)
4. **Wash client's hands.** Have client wash hands with antibacterial soap. Thoroughly dry hands and nails with a sanitized towel.
5. **Do client consultation.** Use the client record/health card to record responses and observations. Check for nail disorders and decide if it is safe and appropriate to perform a service on this client. If the client should not receive service, explain your reasons and refer him or her to a doctor. If you plan to proceed, discuss the service your client wants.

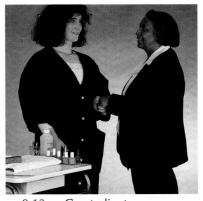

9.12 — Greet client.

6. **Begin manicure.** Begin working with the hand that is **not** the client's favored hand. The favored hand will need to soak longer, because it is used more often. If the client is left-handed, begin with the right hand and if the client is right-handed, begin with the left hand.

WATER MANICURE PROCEDURE

During the manicure, talk with your client about the products and procedures you are using. Suggest products your client will need to maintain the manicure between salon visits. These products might include polish, lotion, top coat, and emery boards.

▶ **NOTE:** The procedure is written for a right-handed client.

1. **Remove polish.** Begin with your client's left hand, little finger. Saturate cotton with polish remover. If your client is wearing artificial nails, use non-acetone remover to avoid damaging them. Hold saturated cotton on nail while you count to ten in your mind. Wipe the old polish off the nail with a stroking motion towards the free edge. If all polish is not removed, repeat this step until all traces of polish are gone. It may be necessary to put cotton around the tip of an orangewood stick and use it to clean polish away from the cuticle area. Repeat this procedure on each finger. (Fig. 9.13)

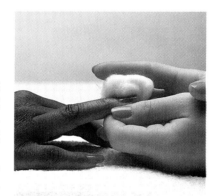

9.13 — Remove polish.

PROCEDURAL TIP

▶ *Roll a piece of cotton between your hands before you use it. This keeps loose cotton fibers from sticking to the nail or finger. An alternative way to remove nail polish is to moisten small pieces of cotton, called **pledgets** (**PLEJ**-ets), with nail polish remover and put them on all the nails at the same time. Pledgets absorb and do not leave a polish smear on the cuticles.*

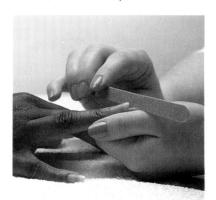

9.14 — Shape nails.

2. **Shape the nails.** Using your emery board or nail file, shape the nails as you and the client have agreed. Start with the left hand, little finger, holding it between your thumb and index finger. Use the coarse side of an emery board to shape the nail. File from the right side to the center of the free edge and from the left side to the center of the free edge. (Fig. 9.14) Do not file into the corners of the nails. (Fig. 9.15) File each hand from the little finger to the thumb.
3. **Soften cuticles.** After filing left hand, put it in your soap bath to soak and soften cuticles while you file the right hand.

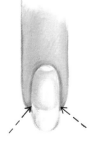

9.15 — Do not file into the corners of the nail.

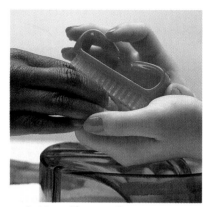

9.16 — Clean nails.

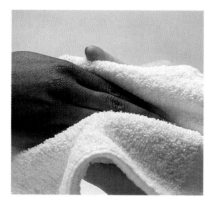

9.17 — Dry hand.

4. **Clean nails.** Brushing nails and hands with a nail brush cleans fingers and pieces of cuticle from the nails. Remove the left hand from the soap bath and brush the fingers with your nail brush. Use downward strokes, starting at the first knuckle and brushing toward the free edge. (Fig. 9.16)

5. **Dry hand.** Dry the hand with the end of a fresh towel. Make sure you dry between the fingers. As you dry, gently push back the cuticle. (Fig. 9.17)

6. **Apply Cuticle Remover.** Use a cotton-tipped orangewood stick to apply cuticle remover to the cuticle of each nail on the hand you've just brushed. (Fig. 9.18) Saturate cotton with cuticle remover and spread generously around cuticles and under the free edge of each finger. This softens and removes cuticle that remains after brushing. Now, put the right hand into the soap bath to soak while you continue to work on your client's left hand. (Fig. 9.19)

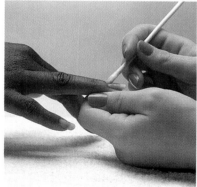
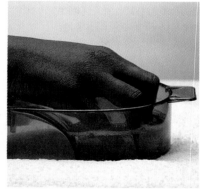

9.18 — Apply cuticle remover.   9.19 — Soak hand.

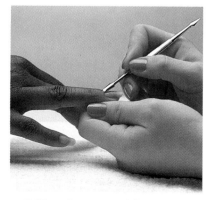

9.20 — Loosen cuticle.

7. **Loosen cuticles.** Use your orangewood stick and/or the spoon end of your steel pusher to gently push back and lift cuticle off of the nails of the left hand. Use a circular movement to help lift cuticles that cling to the nail plate. The cuticle remover will probably remove enough cuticle so that you won't need to clip any. (Fig. 9.20)

8. **Nip cuticles.** Use your cuticle nippers to nip any ragged excess cuticle or hangnails. Try to remove cuticle in one piece. You may need to wipe away excess cuticle remover to see the cuticle

clearly. Be careful not to cut into the mantle, because you will hurt your client. (Fig. 9.21)

> **STATE REGULATION ALERT**
>
> *Some states do not permit nail technicians to nip cuticles or hangnails. Be guided by your instructor.*

9. **Clean under free edge.** Clean under the free edge using a cotton-tipped orangewood stick. Remove right hand from soap bath. Hold left hand over soap bath and brush a last time to remove bits of cuticle and traces of solvent. Then let client rest the left hand on the sanitized towel. (Fig. 9.22)
10. **Repeat steps 4–9 on right hand.**
11. **Bleach nails—optional.** After the filing and cleaning steps, if the client's nails are yellow, you can bleach them with a prepared nail bleach or apply 20 volume (6 percent) hydrogen peroxide. Apply the bleaching agent to the yellowed nail with a cotton-tipped orangewood stick. Be careful not to brush bleach on your client's skin or cuticle, because it will cause irritation. Apply several times if nails are extremely yellow. You may need to bleach certain clients' nails every time you manicure them for a period of time. Since all yellow may not fade after one service, you should plan to repeat the procedure when the client gets the next manicure.
12. **Buff with chamois buffer—optional.** To buff nails, apply dry nail polish to the nail with your orangewood stick. Buff on a diagonal from the base of the nail to its free edge. (Fig. 9.23) Buff in one direction, from left to right with a downward stroke and then from right to left with a downward stroke, forming an "X" pattern. (Fig. 9.24) As you buff, lift the back of the

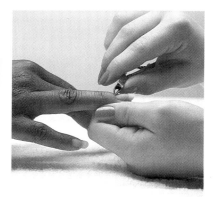

9.21 — Nip cuticles.

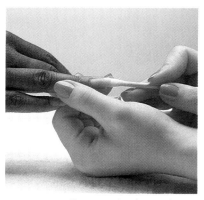

9.22 — Clean under free edge.

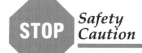 **Safety Caution**

When the cuticle is difficult to push back, be careful not to apply too much pressure at the base of the nail because it could damage the matrix.

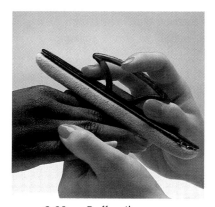

9.23 — Buff nail.

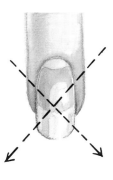

9.24 — Buff nail in an "X" pattern with downward strokes.

buffer off the nail to prevent friction that can cause your client to experience a burning sensation. After buffing, client should wash hands to remove any traces of abrasive or dry polish. The chamois buffer can also be used to smooth out wavy ridges or corrugated nails.

PROCEDURAL TIP

▶ *You may want to spray your client's nail with water before buffing to reduce the heat generated during buffing.*

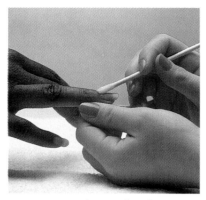
9.25 — Apply cuticle oil.

13. **Apply cuticle oil.** Use a cotton-tipped orangewood stick to apply cuticle oil to each nail. Start with the little finger, left hand, and rub oil into each cuticle in a circular motion. (Fig. 9.25)

14. **Bevel nails.** To bevel (**BEH**-vel) the underside of the free edge, hold emery board at a 45° angle, and file with an upward stroke. This removes any rough edges or cuticle particles. (Fig. 9.26)

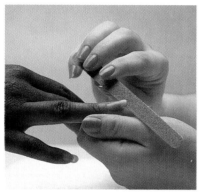
9.26 — Bevel nail.

15. **Apply hand lotion and massage hand and arm.** As a pleasant touch to your manicure before you apply polish, you can treat your client to a hand massage. Apply lotion or cream to the hand and arm with a sanitary spatula. (Follow the procedure for hand and arm massage on pages 116–119.)

16. **Remove traces of oil.** You must remove traces of oil from the nail so the polish will adhere better. Use a small piece of cotton saturated with alcohol or polish remover, and wipe off the nail.

17. **Choose a color.** If your client is undecided about the color of the nail polish, help her choose one. Suggest a shade that complements the skin tone. If the manicure and polish are for a special occasion, pick a color that matches the client's clothing. Generally, darker shades are appropriate for fall and winter and lighter shades are better for spring and summer. Always have a variety of nail polish colors available. Before applying polish, you may ask your client to pay for the service, put on any sweater or jacket, and get out car keys. This will avoid smudges to the fresh polish.

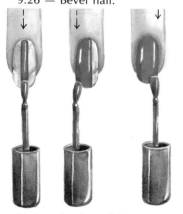
9.27 — Apply polish.

18. **Apply polish.** Polish is applied in four or five coats. The first, the base coat, is followed by two coats of color and one or two applications of top coat. (Fig. 9.27) Roll the polish in your palms to mix. Never shake your polish. Shaking causes air bubbles to form, which will make the polish application rough.

- **Base coat.** Base coat is applied first to keep polish from staining the nails and to help colored polish adhere to the nail. The base coat will stay tacky to the touch. To apply the base coat, take the brush out of the bottle and wipe one side on the neck of the bottle. You should have a bead of polish on the end of the brush. Start in the center of the nail, position brush 1/16 inch away from the cuticle, and brush toward free edge. Using the same technique, do left side of nail, then right side. You should have enough polish on the brush to complete three strokes without having to dip the brush into the polish bottle. If you go back and dab at any spots you missed, the polish will not appear smooth on the nail. The more strokes you make, the more lines or lumps you will have on the client's nail. If you miss a small area on the first color coat, you can cover it on the second coat.
- **Colored polish.** Apply two coats of colored polish with the same technique used for the base coat. Complete your first color coat on both hands before starting the second coat. If you get polish on the cuticle, use a cotton-tipped orangewood stick saturated with polish remover to clean it off. Never use a polish corrector pen because it is unsanitary.
- **Top coat.** Apply one or two coats of top coat to prevent chipping and to give nails a glossy look.
- **Instant nail dry–optional.** Apply instant nail dry on each nail to prevent smudging and dulling.

PROCEDURAL TIP

▶ *If you use an electric nail dryer, put one of your client's hands in the dryer while you polish the other. Put setting on cool; this helps to dry polish surface and make it less likely to smudge.*

Five Types of Polish Application

You have learned how to apply polish correctly to a fingernail. You can create the five types of polished nails listed below:

1. **Full Coverage.** Entire nail plate is polished.
2. **Free edge.** The free edge of the nail is unpolished. This helps to prevent polish from chipping.
3. **Hairline tip.** The nail plate is polished and 1/16 inch is removed from the free edge. This prevents polish from chipping.
4. **Slimline or free walls.** Leave 1/16 inch margin on each side of nail plate. This makes a wide nail appear narrow.

5. **Half moon or lunula.** A half moon shape, the lunula, at the base of the nail is unpolished. (Fig. 9.28)

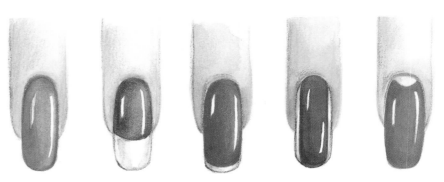

9.28 — Five polish options: full coverage; free edge; hair line tip; slim line or free wall; half moon or lunula

PROCEDURAL TIP

▶ *If you smudge on a finished nail, apply polish remover to the smudge before you put polish on again.*

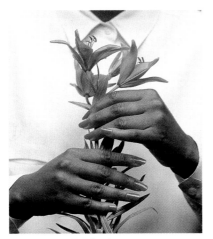

9.29 — Finished water manicure

WATER MANICURE POST-SERVICE

Your water manicure is complete. Follow the post-service procedure described below. (Fig. 9.29)

1. **Make another appointment.** Schedule another appointment with your client to maintain the manicure or to perform another service.

2. **Sell retail products.** Suggest that your client buy products you have discussed during the manicure. Polish, lotion, top coat, etc. are valuable tools for maintaining the nails between salon visits.

3. **Clean up around your table.** Take the time to restore the basic set-up of your table.

4. **Discard used materials.** Place all used materials in the plastic bag at the side of the table. If the bag is full or contains used materials from artificial nail services, discard it in a closed pail.

5. **Sanitize table and implements.** Perform the complete pre-service sanitation procedure. Implements must be sanitized for 20 minutes before they can be used on the next client.

French Manicure

A French manicure is a clean and natural polish application that is very popular in summer months and for weddings. It is also a great base for nail art. You can create endless artistic designs with pearls, rhinestones, and silver striping tapes.

1. **Apply base coat.** Follow the water manicure procedure through the application of base coat. Apply a base coat to the nail as you learned in the water manicure. The base coat can be applied under the free edge as well.
2. **Apply white polish.** Apply white polish to the free edge by starting at one side (usually left side of nail) and sweeping across toward the center of the free edge on a diagonal line. Repeat this on the right side of the nail. This will form a "V" shape. Some clients like this look. If not, fill the open top of the "V," so that you have an even line across the free edge. White may be applied under the free edge. (Figs. 9.30, 9.31, 9.32)

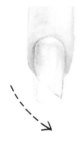

9.30 — Apply white polish on free edge from the left side of the nail to the center.

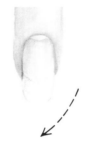

9.31 — Apply white polish on free edge from the right side of the nail to the center.

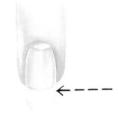

9.32 — Fill in "V" with white polish.

3. **Apply sheer pink, natural, or peach polish.** Apply a sheer pink, natural, or peach color polish from the base to the free edge. Be careful not to get any on the cuticle. Most clients will prefer a pink shade, but choose the color according to skin tone and client preference.
4. **Apply top coat.** Apply a top coat over the entire nail plate and under the free edge if you chose to put it under the free edge previously. (Fig. 9.33)

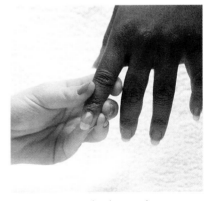

9.33 — Finished French manicure

Reconditioning Hot Oil Manicure

A reconditioning hot oil manicure is of particular benefit to clients who have ridged and brittle nails or dry cuticles. It also improves the hands because it leaves the skin soft. A reconditioning hot oil manicure is recommended once a week. It will add moisture to skin and nails. The oil manicure is especially recommended for a nail biter, because it keeps rough cuticles or hangnails soft.

SUPPLIES

In addition to your standard table set-up, you will need the following items:

1. **Hot oil heater.** This electric heater is used for immersing the client's fingers in the hot oil or cream.
2. **Plastic cups to put in heater.** Most hot oil heaters are made to hold a round or kidney-shaped disposable cup that is filled with the lotion, cream, or oil. This cup comes in multiple packs and should be discarded after each manicure.
3. **Oil for the heater.** Most nail technicians use an oil or cream that is specially prepared for the hot oil heater. Olive oil or hand lotion can also be used. In this procedure, all of these items are referred to as lotion.

RECONDITIONING HOT OIL MANICURE PRE-SERVICE

1. **Do your Pre-service Sanitation Procedure.**
2. **Set up table.** Set up your standard manicuring table, hot oil heater with plastic cup, and lotion
3. **Prepare heater.** Pour lotion into a disposable cup and place it in the heater.
4. **Preheat lotion.** Preheat lotion for 10-15 minutes before seating your client to begin your manicure.
5. **Greet client.**
6. **Wash client's hands.** Have client wash hands with antibacterial soap. Dry hands thoroughly with a fresh towel.
7. **Do client consultation.**
8. **Begin manicure.** Begin working with the hand that is **not** the client's favored hand.

RECONDITIONING HOT OIL MANICURE PROCEDURE

During the procedure talk with your client about the products needed to maintain the manicure between salon visits.

1. **Remove old polish.**
2. **Shape nails.** Shape the nails on the hand that is not the client's favored hand.
3. **Put fingertips in hot lotion.** After shaping the nails on one hand, put it in the hot lotion and file the other hand. (Fig. 9.34)

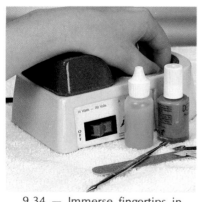

9.34 — Immerse fingertips in hot lotion.

4. **Distribute lotion.** When you remove one hand from the lotion, place the other hand in the lotion. Spread lotion on the hand and arm to the elbow. This will give you enough lotion for the massage. If you run out of lotion, use your spatula to dip more out of the heater and apply it to the hand or arm where needed.
5. **Proceed with hand and arm massage.** Follow the procedure for hand and arm massage described on pages 116–119.
6. **Loosen cuticles.** Use orangewood stick to gently push back cuticles.
7. **Nip cuticles.** Use nippers to nip excess cuticle, if permitted in your state. Let client rest hand on sanitized towel.
8. **Repeat on other hand.** Distribute lotion on the other hand. Proceed with steps 5–7.
9. **Wipe or wash hands.** If necessary, take a warm terry towel and wipe off excess lotion, or have client wash hands.
10. **Apply cold towel.** Close pores on arm and hand with a cold towel. Wrap towel around arm and hand and gently press.
11. **Remove traces of oil.** Saturate cotton in alcohol or polish remover and wipe oil from nails.
12. **Apply polish.**
13. **Complete Manicure Post-Service.** Discard the plastic cup from the hot oil heater.
14. **Sanitize heater.** Use alcohol to prepare the hot oil heater for the next client.

Man's Manicure

A man's manicure is basically the same as a woman's manicure. Table set-up will be the same, except that color polish will not be used. Some men will like a clear liquid polish, and others will prefer a dry polish with your chamois buffer. Using hand cream or lotion is optional. (Fig. 9.35)

PROCEDURE

During the procedure, talk with your client about products that will help him maintain the manicure between visits. You might suggest clear polish and hand cream.

1. **Complete Manicure Pre-Service.**
2. **Remove old polish.** If the client has clear polish from a previous manicure, it must be removed. Begin with his left hand, little finger.

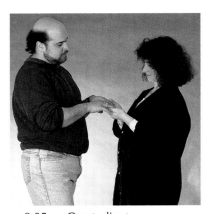

9.35 — Greet client.

112   PART III   BASIC PROCEDURES

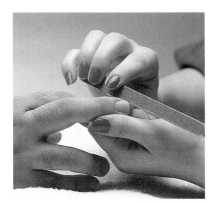

9.36 — Shape nails.

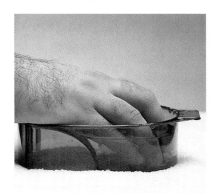

9.37 — Soften cuticles.

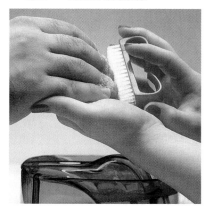

9.38 — Clean nails.

3. **Shape the nails.** Using your emery board or nail file, shape the nails. Start with the left hand, little finger, holding it between your thumb and index finger. You probably won't have much to file; most men keep their nails short. If nails are long, clip them with fingernail clippers before you file. (Fig. 9.36)

PROCEDURAL TIP

▶ *Never file nails that have been soaking. Soaking makes nails soft and easy to break or split when filed.*

4. **Soften cuticles.** After filing left hand, put it in your soap bath to soak and soften cuticles while you file the right hand. (Fig. 9.37)

5. **Clean nails and hands.** Brushing hands and nails with the nail brush cleans fingers and pieces of cuticle from nails. Remove left hand from the soap bath and brush the fingers with your nail brush in downward strokes, starting at the first knuckle and brushing in one direction toward the free edge. (Fig. 9.38)

6. **Dry hand.** Dry the hand with the end of the towel that is wrapped around the cushion. Make sure you dry between the fingers. As you dry, gently push back the cuticle. (Fig. 9.39)

7. **Apply cuticle remover.** Use a cotton-tipped orangewood stick to apply cuticle remover to the back of each nail on the hand you've just brushed. Now, put the right hand into the soap bath to soak while you continue to work on your client's left hand. (Fig. 9.40)

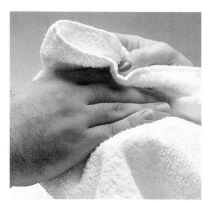

9.39 — Dry hand.

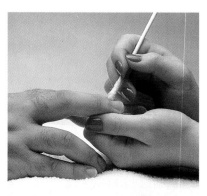

9.40 — Apply cuticle remover.

8. **Loosen cuticles.** Most men will need more work done on their cuticles, as they will generally have more cuticle than women. Women tend to push their own cuticles back between appointments, whereas men don't. Use pusher to gently push back and lift cuticle off of the nails of the left hand. (Fig. 9.41)

9. **Nip cuticles.** If you have to nip excess cuticle or hangnails, try to do so in one piece. (Fig. 9.42)

10. **Clean under free edge.** Clean under the free edge with a cotton-tipped orangewood stick. Hold left hand over soap bath and brush a last time to remove bits of cuticle and traces of solvent that remain on the nail. Then let client put the left hand on a sanitized towel. (Fig. 9.43)

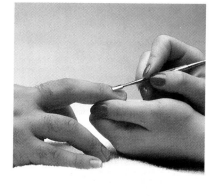

9.41 — Loosen cuticle with pusher.

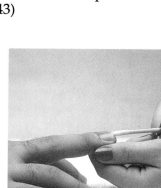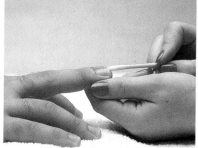

9.42 — Nip cuticles.   9.43 — Clean under free edge.

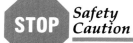

Safety Caution

Be sure to have styptic powder (powdered alum) on hand in case of minor bleeding.

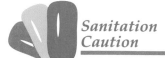

Sanitation Caution

The cotton on your orangewood stick needs to be changed after each use.

11. **Repeat steps 5–10 on right hand.**

12. **Bleach nails—optional.** If the client's nails are yellow you can bleach them with a prepared nail bleach or by applying 20 volume (6 percent) hydrogen peroxide.

13. **Buff with chamois buffer.** If you and your client wish, you can buff nails at this point. To shine nails, apply dry nail polish to the nail with your orangewood stick, buffing on a diagonal from the base of the nail to its free edge. Buff in one direction, from left to right, with a downward stroke and cross over from right to left with a downward stroke, forming an "X" pattern. As you buff, lift the back of the buffer off the nail to prevent friction that can cause your client to experience a burning sensation on the nail. After buffing, client should wash hands to remove any traces of abrasive or dry polish. The chamois buffer can also be used to smooth out wavy ridges or corrugated nails. This is done with an abrasive, such as pumice powder, which is applied to the nail with an orangewood stick. (Fig. 9.44)

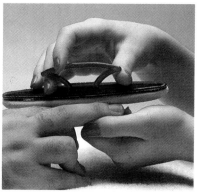

9.44 — Buff nails with chamois buffer.

114 PART III BASIC PROCEDURES

> ### STATE REGULATION ALERT
> *Some states do not permit the use of a chamois buffer. If they do, chamois must be changed for each client. Be guided by your instructor.*

14. **Apply cuticle oil.** Use a cotton-tipped orangewood stick to apply cuticle oil to each nail. Start with the little finger, left hand and rub oil into each cuticle in a circular motion. (Fig. 9.45)

15. **Bevel nails.** To bevel the underside of the free edge, hold emery board at a 45° angle, and file with an upward stroke. This removes any rough edges or cuticle particles.

16. **Apply hand lotion and massage hand and arm—optional.** As a pleasant touch to your manicure before you apply polish, you can treat your client to a hand lotion or hand cream massage. Apply lotion or cream to the arm and hand with a sanitary spatula. (Follow the procedure for hand and arm massage on pages 116–119.) (Fig. 9.46)

17. **Remove traces of oil.** Remove traces of oil by using a small piece of cotton that has been saturated with alcohol or polish remover. Wipe off the nail to allow polish to adhere better.

18. **Polish nails.** If your client wants polish, apply a base coat and a clear top coat. Follow with instant nail dry. (Fig. 9.47)

19. **Complete Manicure Post-Service Procedure.**

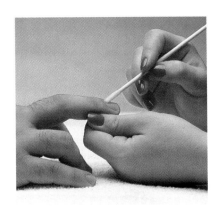

9.45 — Apply cuticle oil.

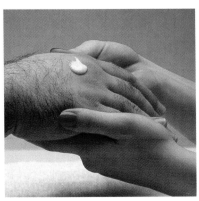

9.46 — Apply hand lotion.

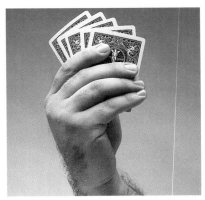

9.47 — Finished man's manicure

Moving Men Into Manicuring

Men love manicures, too, once you get them to try this service. How do you do that? Technicians who have a significant percentage of male clients say the best way is to hold a men's night in the salon. Place an ad in the business or sports section of your local paper or have students pass out flyers to men, announcing the special evening. Stress your men's high-buff manicure or sports pedicure with foot massage and they'll get the idea. Avoid an overly feminine atmosphere in your nail area. Instead, strive for a clean, clinical atmosphere. Include men's magazines in your waiting area and create male-oriented displays of files, buffers, and callus removers, positioned slightly away from polishes.

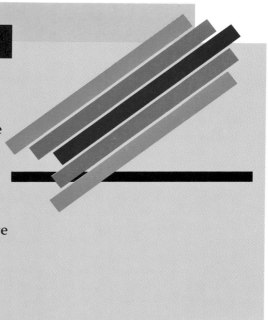

Electric Manicure

The electric manicure is given with a small portable machine with a motor. The electric manicure tool looks like a portable drill. It uses a variety of attachments that include an emery wheel, cuticle pusher, brush, and nail buffing disk.

Before using an electric manicure machine, read the manufacturer's instructions carefully. State regulations on this procedure may vary.

Care should be taken with the attachments. Do not apply too much pressure at the base of the nail with the cuticle pusher and buffer. Do not hold in one spot because it will cause a burning sensation.

The emery wheel or nail shaper is like your emery board. It has a coarse side and a fine side. The cuticle pusher is like your steel pusher. It is used to push back excess cuticle. The nail brush is like the nail brush used in a water manicure. It is used to remove small bits of cuticle and to cleanse the nail. The buffing disc works like your chamois buffer. It is used to smooth corrugations and add shine to the nail. Be careful when you use the buffer because it causes a burning sensation on the nail if you apply too much pressure. Be sure to lift it frequently to prevent this or mist the nail with water before buffing.

Your electric manicure machine may include a callus remover disc. It is much coarser than the emery disc and is shaped like a cylinder. Use it around tip of finger or at the side to remove callus growth.

STATE REGULATION ALERT

Some states do not permit the use of an electric manicure machine. Be guided by your instructor.

Hand and Arm Massage

Massage is a service that can be offered with any type of manicure. Massaging stimulates blood flow, and is relaxing to the client.

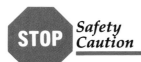
Safety Caution

DO NOT massage if client has high blood pressure, heart condition, or has had a stroke. Massage increases circulation and may be harmful to this client. Have client consult a physician first. Be very careful to avoid vigorous massage of joints if your client has arthritis. Talk with your client throughout the massage and adjust your touch to the client's needs.

HAND MASSAGE TECHNIQUES

1. **Relaxer movement.** This is a form of massage known as "joint movement." At the beginning of the hand massage the client has already received hand lotion or cream. Place client's elbow on cushion. With one hand, brace client's arm. With your other hand, hold client's wrist and bend it back and forth slowly, about five to ten times, until you feel the client has relaxed. (Fig. 9.48)

2. **Joint movement on fingers.** Bring client's arm down, brace the arm with the left hand, and with your right hand start with the little finger, holding it at the base of the nail. Gently rotate fingers to form circles. Work towards the thumb, about 3–5 times on each finger. (Fig. 9.49)

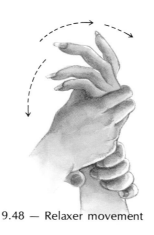

9.48 — Relaxer movement

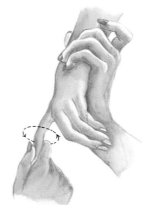

9.49 — Joint movement on fingers

3. **Circular movement in palm.** This is "effleurage" (**EF**-loo-rahzh)—light stroking that relaxes and soothes. Place client's elbow on the cushion and, with your thumbs in the client's palm, rotate in a circular movement in opposite directions. (Fig. 9.50)

4. **Circular movement on wrist.** Hold client's hand with both of your hands, placing your thumbs on top of client's hand, your fingers below the hand. Move your thumbs in a circular movement in opposite directions from the client's wrist to the knuckle on back of the client's hand. Move up and down, 3–5 times. The last time you rotate up, wring the client's wrist by bracing your hands around the wrist and gently twisting in opposite directions. This is a form of friction massage movement that is a deep rubbing action and very stimulating. (Fig. 9.51)

5. **Circular movement on back of hand and fingers.** Now rotate down the back of the client's hand using your thumbs. Rotate down the little finger and the client's thumb and gently squeeze off at the tips of client's fingers. Go back and rotate down the ring finger and index finger, gently squeezing off. Now do the middle finger and squeeze off at tip. This restores blood flow to normal. (Fig. 9.52)

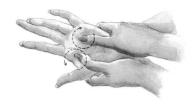

9.50 — Circular movement "Effleurage"

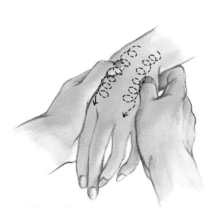

9.51 — Circular movement on wrist

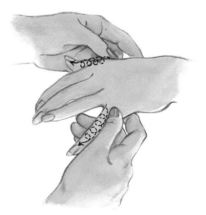

9.52 — Circular movement on back of hand and fingers

ARM MASSAGE TECHNIQUES

1. **Distribute cream or lotion.** Apply a small amount of cream to the client's arm and work it in. Work from the client's wrist toward the elbow, except on the last movement; work from the elbow to wrist, then squeeze off at fingertips, as you did at the end of hand massage. Apply more cream if necessary.

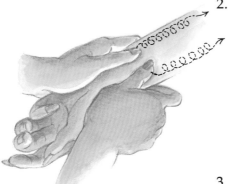

9.53 — Effleurage on arms

2. **Effleurage on arms.** Put client's arm down on the table, bracing the arm with your hands. Hold your client's hand palm up in your hand. Your fingers should be under the client's hand; your thumbs side-by-side in your client's palm. Rotate your thumbs in opposite directions, starting at the client's wrist and working towards the elbow. When you reach the elbow, slide your hand down client's arm to the wrist and rotate back up to the elbow 3–5 times. Turn client's arm over and repeat 3–5 times on the top side of arm. (Fig. 9.53)

3. **Wringing movement on arm**—*friction massage movement.* A friction massage involves deep rubbing to the muscles. Bend client's elbow so the arm is horizontal in front of you, with the back of the hand facing up. Place your hands around the arm with your fingers facing the same direction as the arm, and gently twist in opposite directions as you would wring out a washcloth, from wrist to elbow. Do this up and down the forearm 3–5 times. (Fig. 9.54)

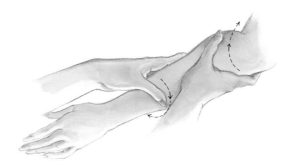

9.54 — Wringing movement on arm friction massage

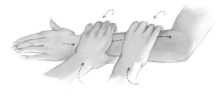

9.55 — Kneading movement on arm

4. **Kneading movement on arm.** This technique is called the **petrissage** (PE-tre-sahza) kneading movement. It is very stimulating and increases blood flow. Place your thumbs on the top side of client's arm so they are horizontal. Move them in opposite directions, from wrist to elbow and back down to wrist. This squeezing motion moves flesh over bone and stimulates the arm tissue. Do this 3–5 times. (Fig. 9.55)

5. **Rotation of elbow**—*friction massage movement.* Brace client's arm with your left hand and, with cotton-tipped orangewood stick, apply cream to elbow. Cup elbow with your right hand and rotate your hand over the client's elbow. Do this 3–5 times.

To finish the elbow massage, move your left arm of the client's forearm. Gently slide both hands d forearm from the elbow to the fingertips as if climbing a rope. Repeat this 3–5 times. (Fig. 9.56)

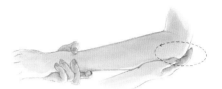

9.56 — Rotation of elbow

Review Questio

1. When you give a manicure, you need equipment, implements, materials, and nail cosmetics. Give three examples of each of these manicuring supplies.
2. What are two reasons for having a manicuring table that is sanitary and properly equipped?
3. Describe the four basic nail shapes.
4. List the six steps in the water manicure pre-service.
5. Briefly describe the water manicure procedure.
6. Name the five types of polish applications.
7. List the five steps in the water manicure post-service.
8. List the four steps in the French manicure procedure.
9. What are the three benefits of the reconditioning hot oil manicure? How often should clients receive a reconditioning hot oil manicure?
10. What type of polish application is included in a man's manicure?
11. Name five hand massage techniques and five arm massage techniques.
12. What are two safety cautions for hand and arm massage?

LEARNING OBJECTIVES

After you have studied this chapter, you should be able to:
1. *Identify the equipment and materials needed for a pedicure and explain what they are used for.*
2. *List the steps in the pedicure pre-service procedure.*
3. *Demonstrate the proper procedures and precautions for a pedicure.*
4. *Describe the proper technique to use in filing toenails.*
5. *Demonstrate your ability to perform foot massage properly.*

The information in this chapter will show you the pedicuring skills you need to care for clients' feet, toes, and toenails. A **pedicure** includes trimming, shaping, and polishing toenails as well as foot massage. Pedicures are a standard service performed by nail technicians. They are a basic part of good foot care for any client and they are particularly important for clients before summer beach visits. Proper foot care through pedicuring improves both personal appearance and basic foot comfort.

PROCEDURAL TIP

▶ When making an appointment for a pedicure, suggest that your client wear open-toe shoes or sandals so that polish will not smear. Also remind your client that hose will need to be removed before the pedicure can be performed.

Pedicure Supplies

You will need to have the following supplies in addition to your standard manicure set-up to perform pedicures: (Figs. 10.1, 10.2)

Pedicuring station. A station includes a chair for the client, a footrest for the client, and a chair for the nail technician. Pedicure stations that combine all these items into one piece of furniture are available.

Pedicuring stool and footrest. A pedicuring stool is a low stool that will make it easier for you to work on your client's feet. Some pedicuring stools come with a footrest for the client, or a separate footrest can be used.

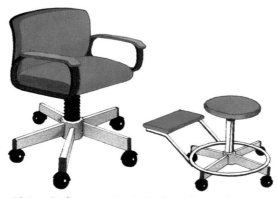

10.1 — Pedicure station including client's chair, footrest, and pedicuring stool

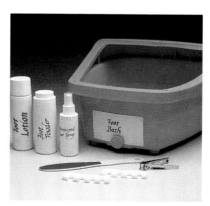

10.2 — Supplies needed for pedicure

air. The client's chair should be comfortable with arm

soap baths. These pedicure baths are filled with warm
ntibacterial soap in which to soak the client's feet. The
 e large enough to immerse the client's feet. You will
 asins, one for warm water with soap or detergent and
 erial agent and the other for rinse water.

rators. Foam rubber toe separators or cotton used to keep
 during the pedicure.

 . Used to remove dry skin or **callus** growths.

clippers. Two types of toenail clippers are available; both
 table for a professional pedicure.

tic foot spray. Contains an **antifungal** (an-ti-**FUN**-gahl)
 well as a mild antiseptic.

cterial soap. Antibacterial (an-ti-bak-**TEER**-ee-ahl) soap for
pedicuring contains a soap or detergent, an antifungal agent, and
an antibacterial agent.

Foot lotion. Used during foot massage. Hand lotion can also be used.

Foot powder. Contains an antifungal agent for keeping feet dry after pedicure.

Pedicure slippers. These sanitized plastic or disposable paper slippers are optional.

Pedicure

As with other procedures, a pedicure involves three parts: the Pre-Service, the Pedicure Procedure, and the Post-Service. In the Pre-Service you will sanitize your implements, greet your client, and do a client consultation. Next you will do the steps involved in the actual procedure. Then, in the Post-Service, you will schedule another appointment for your client, sell the retail products you discussed during the service, and sanitize.

PEDICURE PRE-SERVICE

Your pedicure area should be close to a sink so it is convenient when you fill the pedicure baths with water.

1. Complete your pre-service sanitation procedure. (This procedure is described on pages 29–30.)
2. Your station should be set up to include a pedicuring stool, client's chair, and a footrest for your client.
3. Spread one terry cloth towel on the floor in front of client's chair to put feet on during the pedicure. Put another towel over the stool to dry feet.

4. Set up your standard manicuring table in your pedicuring station. Add toe separators, foot file, toenail clippers, antiseptic antifungal foot spray, antibacterial soap, foot lotion, foot powder, and pedicure slippers to your table.

5. Fill both basins with warm water. Add a measured amount of antibacterial soap to the bath (follow manufacturer's directions). Add a few drops of antiseptic to the other bath for rinsing. Put baths in front of towel on the floor.

6. Greet client.

7. Complete client consultation. Use client record/health card to record responses and observations. Check for nail disorders and decide if it is safe and appropriate to perform a service on your client. If infection or inflammation is present, refer your client to a physician. If athlete's foot is present, you may not perform a pedicure.

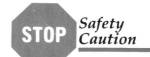

Safety Caution

Be sure the floor around pedicure area is dry because wet floors are slippery and you or your clients can fall. When water is spilled, wipe it up immediately.

PEDICURE PROCEDURE

During the procedure, talk with your client about the products that are needed to maintain the service between salon visits. You might suggest polish, top coat, foot lotion, and foot powder.

1. **Remove shoes and socks.** Ask your client to remove shoes, socks, and hose and roll pant legs to the knees.
2. **Spray feet.** Spray feet with foot spray or wipe them with antiseptic. (Fig. 10.3)
3. **Soak feet.** Put client's feet in soap bath for 5–10 minutes to wash and sanitize the feet before you begin the pedicure. (Fig. 10.4)
4. **Rinse feet.** Remove both feet from soap bath and rinse in rinse bath.

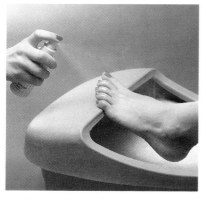
10.3 — Spray feet.

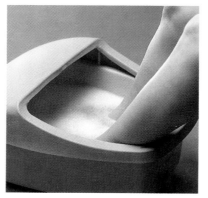
10.4 — Soak feet.

PART III BASIC PROCEDURES

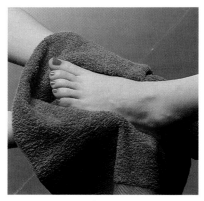

10.5 — Dry feet.

5. **Dry feet.** Take one foot out of the rinse water and dry it off. Make sure you dry between the toes. Remove other foot from rinse bath and thoroughly dry. Ask client to place both feet on the towel you have placed on the floor. (Fig. 10.5)
6. **Remove polish.** Remove polish from little toe on left foot, working towards big toe. Repeat with the right foot. (Fig. 10.6)
7. **Clip nails.** Clip the toenails of the left foot so that they are even with the end of the toe. (Fig. 10.7)

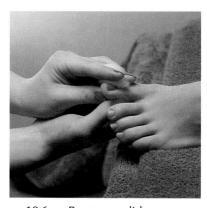

10.6 — Remove polish.

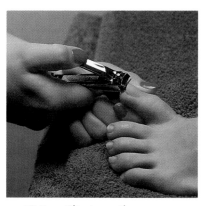

10.7 — Clip toenails.

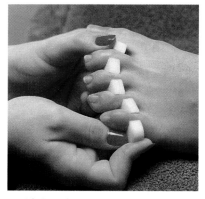

10.8 — Insert toe separators.

8. **Insert toe separators.** Use both hands to carefully insert toe separators or cotton between the toes of the left foot. (Fig. 10.8)
9. **File nails.** File the nails of the left foot with an emery board. File them straight across, rounding them slightly at the corners to conform to the shape of the toes. To avoid ingrown toenails, do not file into the corners of the nails. Smooth rough edges with the fine side of an emery board. (Fig. 10.9)
10. **Use foot file.** Use foot file on ball and heel of foot to remove dry skin and callus growths. Do not file too much because it can cause irritation and bleeding. (Fig. 10.10)

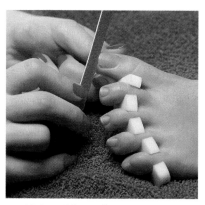

10.9 — File nails.

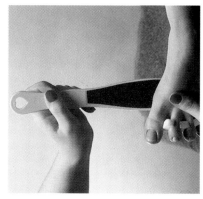

10.10 — Use foot file.

> **STATE REGULATION ALERT**
>
> *A credo knife is a holder that supports a razor blade. Some states do not allow the use of the credo knife to remove callus growths because it can easily cut the client's foot. Be guided by your instructor about the use of a credo knife in your state.*

11. **Rinse foot.** Remove toe separators and place left foot in foot bath.
12. **Repeat steps 7–11 on right foot.**
13. **Brush nails.** Remove left foot from foot bath and brush nails with nail brush. Rinse foot in rinse bath and dry thoroughly. Insert toe separators or cotton between toes. (Fig. 10.11)
14. **Apply cuticle solvent.** Use cotton-tipped orangewood stick to apply cuticle solvent to left foot. Begin with the little toe and work towards the big toe. You may apply solvent under free edge as well to soften excess skin beneath it. (Fig. 10.12)
15. **Push back cuticle.** On left foot, gently push cuticles with orangewood stick. If cuticle clipping is permitted in your state, clip only to remove a hangnail. (Fig. 10.13)

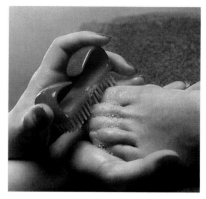
10.11 — Brush nails.

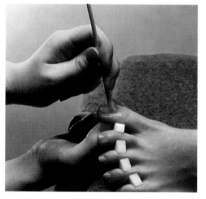
10.12 — Apply cuticle solvent.

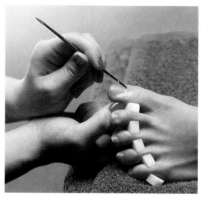
10.13 — Push back cuticle.

16. **Brush foot.** Remove toe separators. Ask your client to dip left foot into soap bath. With the left foot over the soap bath, brush with nail brush to remove bits of cuticle and solvent. Rinse foot in rinse bath and dry thoroughly. Place foot on towel.
17. **Apply lotion.** Apply lotion to foot for massage. Use a firm touch to avoid tickling your client's feet. (Fig. 10.14)
18. **Massage foot.** Perform foot massage on the left foot. Then place foot on a clean towel on the floor. (See Massage techniques on pages 127–129.)

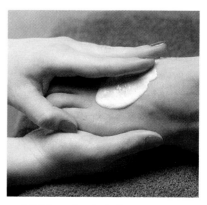
10.14 — Apply lotion.

19. **Proceed with steps 13–19 on the right foot.**
20. **Remove traces of lotion.** Remove traces of lotion from toenails of both feet with a small piece of cotton that has been saturated with polish remover.
21. **Apply polish.** Reinsert the toe separators. Apply base coat, two coats of color, and top coat to toenails. Spray with instant nail dry. Place feet on a towel to dry.
22. **Powder feet.** When polish is dry, power feet before the client puts shoes on.

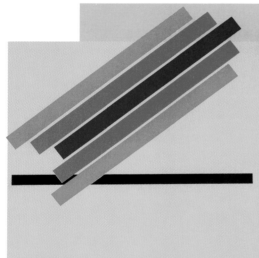

Winter Wonders

It's only human nature that clients ignore their feet in the winter, when they're concealed, and rush in for a pedicure when the sandals come out. To maintain a steady flow of clients in your pedicure area year round, pair on-going education with your winter promotions. For example, offer a mid-winter, pick-me-up pedicure, a winter exfoliating treatment to remove dead skin cells on feet that rarely come out of socks, or a special on dry skin treatment for feet. They're the same services you offer all year, with a new promotional slant.

PEDICURE POST-SERVICE

Your pedicure is now complete. Follow the post-service procedure described below. (Fig. 10.15)

1. **Make another appointment.** Schedule another pedicure appointment for your client.
2. **Advise client.** Advise client about proper foot care. Remind client that wearing tight shoes and very high heels can cause ingrown toenails.
3. **Sell retail products.** Suggest that your client buy products you have discussed during the pedicure. Products such as polish, lotion, and top coat help to maintain the pedicure.
4. **Clean pedicure area.** Dump out basins and wipe them with alcohol to sanitize. Dry basins and put them away. Wipe table and footrest with alcohol.

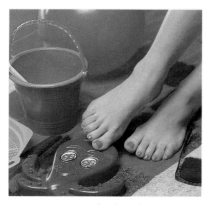

10.15 — Finished pedicure

5. **Discard used materials.** Place all used materials in the plas[tic] bag at the side of the table. If the bag is full, discard it i[n a] closed pail.
6. **Sanitize table and implements.** Perform the complete service sanitation procedure. In most states this procedure for 20 minutes of proper sanitation before implements ca[n be] used on the next client. Return your table to its basic se[tup.]

Foot massage during a pedicure stimulates blood flow and is relaxing to the client. These techniques and illustrations provide directions for massage of the left foot.

FOOT MASSAGE TECHNIQUES

1. **Relaxer movement to the joints of the foot.** Rest client's foot on footrest or stool. Grasp the leg just above the ankle with your left hand. This will brace the client's leg and foot. Use your right hand to hold left foot just beneath toes and rotate foot in a circular motion. (Fig. 10.16)
2. **Effleurage on top of foot.** Place both thumbs on top of foot at instep. Move your thumbs in circular movements in opposite directions down the center of the top of the foot. Continue this movement to the toes. Keep one hand in contact with foot or leg, slide one hand at a time back firmly to instep and rotate back down to toes. This is a relaxing movement. Repeat 3–5 times. (Fig. 10.17)
3. **Effleurage on heel (bottom of foot).** Use the same thumb movement that you did in the massage technique above. Start at the base of the toes and move from the ball of the foot to the heel, rotating your thumbs in opposite directions. Slide hands back to the top of the foot. This is a relaxing movement. Repeat 3–5 times. (Fig. 10.18)

STOP — Safety Caution

DO NOT massage if client has high blood pressure, heart condition, or has had a stroke. Massage increases circulation and may be harmful to such a client. Have your client consult a physician before receiving a massage.

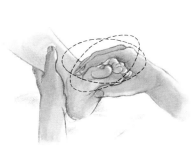

10.16 — Relaxer movement to the joints of the foot

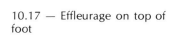

10.17 — Effleurage on top of foot

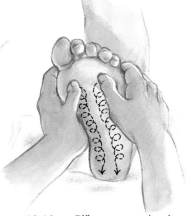

10.18 — Effleurage on heel

4. **Effleurage movement on toes.** Start with the little toe, using thumb on top and index finger on bottom of foot. Hold each toe and rotate with thumb. Start at base of toe and work towards the end of the toes. This is relaxing and soothing. Repeat 3–5 times. (Fig. 10.19)

5. **Joint movement for toes.** Start with the little toe and make a figure eight with each toe. Repeat 3–5 times. (Fig. 10.20)

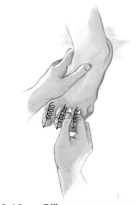
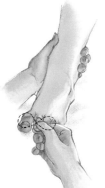

10.19 — Effleurage on toes

10.20 — Joint movement for toes

Safety Caution

If client has had a plantar's wart removed by a podiatrist either chemically or by excision, do not apply thumb compression to that area.

6. **Thumb compression –** *friction movement.* Make a fist with your fingers, keeping your thumb out. Apply firm pressure with your thumb and move your fist up the heel towards the ball of the foot. Work from the left side of foot and back down the right side towards the heel. As you massage over the bottom of the foot, check for any nodules or bumps. If you find one, be very gentle because the area may be tender. This movement stimulates the blood flow and increases circulation. (Fig. 10.21)

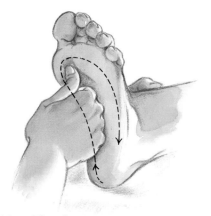

10.21 — Thumb compression "friction movement"

7. **Metatarsal scissors (a petrissage massage movement, kneading).** Place your fingers on top of foot along the metatarsal bones with your thumb underneath the foot. Knead up and down along each bone by raising your thumb and lower fingers to apply pressure. This promotes flexibility and stimulates blood flow. Repeat 3–5 times. (Fig. 10.22)

8. **Fist twist compression (a friction movement, deep rubbing).** Place left hand on top of foot and make a fist with your right hand. Your left hand will apply pressure while your right hand twists around the bottom of the foot. This helps stimulate blood flow. Repeat 3–5 times up and around foot. (Fig. 10.23)

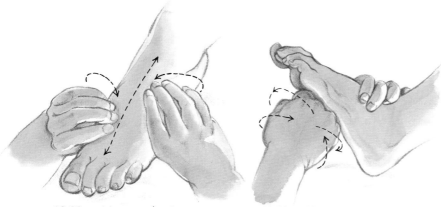

10.22 — Metatarsal scissors   10.23 — Fist twist compression

9. **Effleurage on instep.** Place fingers at ball of foot. Move fingers in circular movements in opposite directions. Massage to end of each toe, gently squeezing the tip of each toe. (Fig. 10.24)

10. **Percussion or tapotement movement.** Use fingertips to perform percussion or tapotement (tah-**POT**-mynt) movements to lightly tap over the entire foot to reduce blood circulation and complete massage.

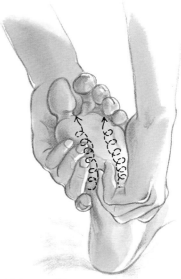

10.24 — Effleurage on instep

Review Questions

1. Name five pedicure supplies.
2. List the eight steps in the pedicure pre-service.
3. Briefly describe the pedicure procedure.
4. Describe the proper technique to use in filing toenails.
5. List the six steps in the pedicure post-service.
6. Name six foot massage techniques.
7. What is a safety caution for pedicuring?

PART IV

THE ART OF NAIL TECHNOLOGY

- *Chapter 11 - Nail Tips*
- *Chapter 12 - Nail Wraps*
- *Chapter 13 - Acrylic Nails*
- *Chapter 14 - The Creative Touch*

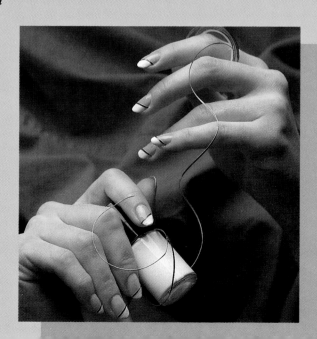

CHAPTER 11

Nail Tips

LEARNING OBJECTIVES

After you have studied this chapter, you should be able to:
1. Identify the supplies needed for nail tips and explain what they are used for.
2. Identify the two types of nail tips.
3. Demonstrate the proper procedure and precautions to use in applying nail tips.
4. Describe the proper maintenance of tips.
5. Demonstrate the proper removal of tips.

Introduction

A *nail tip* is an artificial nail made of plastic, nylon, or acetate. Tips are adhered to the natural nail to add extra length. Usually tips are combined with another artificial service, such as a fabric wrap or sculptured nail, since a tip worn with no overlay is very weak. If a client chooses to wear a tip with no overlay, the tip is considered a temporary service.

Supplies for Nail Tips

In addition to the materials on your basic manicuring table, you will need the following supplies for nail tip application. (Fig. 11.1)

Abrasive. A rough surface that is used to shape or smooth the nail and remove the shine. It usually looks like a large emery board or disk, but it can be any shape or color.

Buffer block. Lightweight rectangular block that is abrasive and used to buff nails.

Nail adhesive. Glue or bonding agent used to secure the nail tip to the natural nail. It usually comes in a tube with a pointed applicator tip or one-drop applicator.

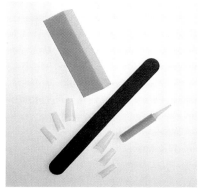

11.1 — Supplies needed for tip application

Nail tips. All tips have a *well* that serves as the point of contact with the nail plate. The position stop is the point where the nail plate meets the tip before it is glued to the nail. Tips are designed with either a partial or full *well*. (Fig. 11.2) The tip should never cover more than 1/2 of the natural nail plate. Tips come in large boxes that have an assortment of sizes. Some nail technicians prefer to have tips from several different manufacturers, since they vary slightly in size and shape. With a wide assortment, it is easier to fit each client with precisely the right size and shape tip.

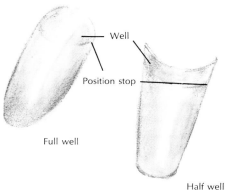

11.2 — Tip with half well and tip with full well

Nail Tip Application

NAIL TIP APPLICATION PRE-SERVICE

1. Complete pre-service sanitation procedure. (This procedure is described on pages 29–30.)

2. Set up your standard manicuring table. Add abrasives, buffer blocks, nail adhesive, and nail tips to your table.

3. Greet client and ask her to wash hands with antibacterial soap. Thoroughly dry hands with a fresh towel.

4. Do client consultation, using client record/health card to record responses and observations. Check for nail disorders and decide if it is safe and appropriate to perform a service on this client. If the client should not receive service, explain your reasons and refer her to a doctor.

NAIL TIP APPLICATION PROCEDURE

During the procedure, discuss products such as polish, top coat, and lotion that will help your client maintain the service between salon visits.

1. **Remove old polish.** Begin with your client's left hand, little finger, and work toward the thumb. Then repeat on the right hand.

2. **Push back cuticle.** Use a cotton-tipped orangewood stick to gently push back cuticle. Use a light touch because the cuticle is dry.

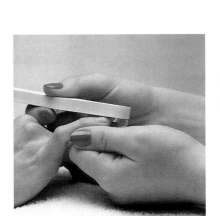

11.3 — Remove shine from nails.

3. **Buff nail to remove shine.** Buff lightly over the nail plate with medium/fine abrasive to remove the natural oil. Do not use a coarse abrasive and be careful not to apply extreme pressure. (Fig. 11.3)

4. **Clean nails.** Ask client to dip nails briefly in fingerbowl filled with antibacterial soap and warm water. Use a nail brush to clean nails while holding them over the fingerbowl. Rinse nails in clear water. (Fig. 11.4) Do not soak client's nails in water before you apply a nail tip. When water is used to rinse the fingers, dip them briefly in fingerbowl. Natural nails are porous and retain water. Water-soaked nails are a perfect breeding ground for mold and fungus under the nail tip.

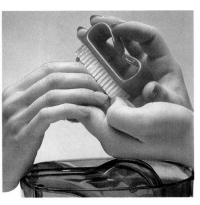

11.4 — Clean nails.

5. **Size tips.** Select the proper size tips. Make sure the tips you choose completely cover the nail plate from sidewall to sidewall but never cover more than half the length of the nail. (Fig. 11.5) Trim tips to the right size if the well covers too much of the nail. Put all sized tips on towel in order of finger size.

6. **Apply nail antiseptic.** Use a cotton-tipped orangewood stick or spray to apply nail antiseptic to nails. Begin with the little finger on the left hand. The antiseptic will remove more of the remaining natural oil and dehydrate the nail for better adhesion. (Fig. 11.6)

7. **Apply adhesive.** Place enough adhesive on nail plate to cover area where tip will be placed. Do not let adhesive run onto the skin. Apply adhesive from the middle of the nail plate to free edge. (Fig. 11.7)

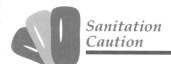

Sanitation Caution

If you accidently touch the nails after you apply antiseptic, you must clean them again and reapply antiseptic.

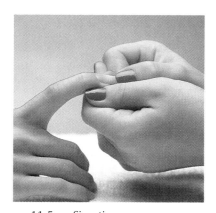
11.5 — Size tips.

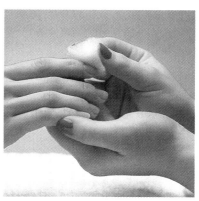
11.6 — Apply nail antiseptic.

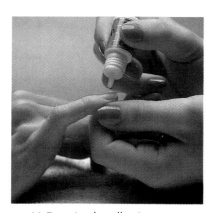
11.7 — Apply adhesive.

PROCEDURAL TIP

▶ *An alternate method of applying adhesive is to apply to the well of the tip. This may ensure that fewer air bubbles are trapped in adhesive.*

8. **Slide on tips.** Slide pre-sized tips on the nails at a 45° angle until the nail hits the position stop. To ensure a secure fit, make sure the tip does not slide past stop. Press firmly for 10 seconds to secure. Check the tip for white spots or air bubbles. If any are present the tip must be reapplied. (Fig. 11.8)

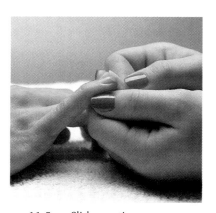
11.8 — Slide on tips.

9. **Apply adhesive bead to seam.** Apply a bead of adhesive to seam between the natural nail plate and the tip to strengthen the stress point. (Fig. 11.9)
10. **Trim nail tip.** Trim the nail tip to desired length using the large nail clippers. Cut from one side, then the other. Cutting the tip straight across causes weakening of the plastic. (Fig. 11.10)

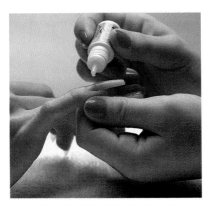

11.9 — Apply adhesive bead to seam.

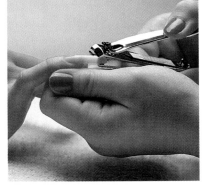

11.10 — Trim nail tip.

11. **Blend tip into natural nail.** Sand the shine off the tip with a semi-coarse abrasive. Make sure you keep the file flat on the nail at all times. Never hold file at an angle because filing at an angle can make a groove in the nail plate. (Fig. 11.11)
12. **Buff tip for perfect blend.** Use the buffer block to gently buff down the area between the natural nail plate and the tip extension. The tip should blend with the natural nail so that there is no visible line or cloudiness between the two. (Fig. 11.12)
13. **Shape nail.** Use abrasive to shape new, longer nail. (Fig. 11.13)

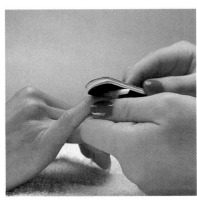

11.11 — Blend tip into natural nail.

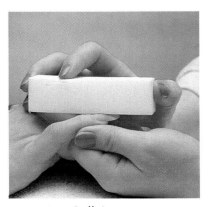

11.12 — Buff tip.

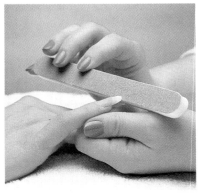

11.13 — Shape tip.

14. **Proceed with desired service.** Your tip application is now complete. Although your client's tips blend perfectly with natural nails, tips are very seldom worn without an additional nail service such as wraps, acrylic nails, or gel nails. You are ready to proceed with the service that your client has chosen. (Fig. 11.14)

NAIL TIP POST-SERVICE

If your client is only wearing tips as a temporary service, add a drop of cuticle oil to each nail and buff.

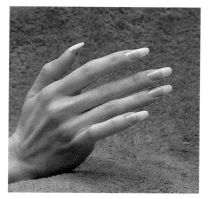

11.14 — Finished tip application

1. **Make another appointment.** Schedule another appointment with your client to remove tips and condition nails and cuticles.

2. **Sell retail products.** Suggest that your client buy products necessary to maintain her nails throughout the week. Polish, lotion, top coat, etc. are valuable maintenance tools for her to have.

3. **Clean up around your table.** Take the time to restore the basic set-up of your table. Cap glue and clean applicator tips in acetone.

4. **Discard used materials.** Place all used materials in the plastic bag at the side of the table. If the bag is full or contains used materials from artificial nail services, discard it in a closed pail.

5. **Sanitize table and implements.** Perform the complete pre-service sanitation procedure. Implements need to be sanitized 20 minutes before they can be used on the next client.

Tips On Selling Tips

Easy does it when it comes to length if your client is trying tips for the first time. If your client has always had short nails, give her tips that are conservative. By cutting back the tips to a manageable length, your client will be able to enjoy the advantages of artificial nails without having to get used to the added length. She will have beautiful, fashionable nails and you will have a satisfied client who may become a regular at your salon.

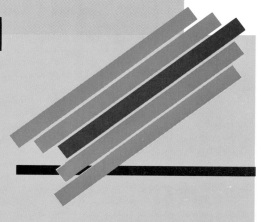

Maintenance and Removal of Tips

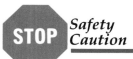
Safety Caution

Never nip off nail tips because you might cause permanent damage to the nail bed.

MAINTENANCE

Clients wearing tips will need weekly or biweekly manicures for regluing and rebuffing. Reglue at the seam between the natural nail and the tip. Most tips need non-acetone polish remover because acetone remover dissolves the tips.

TIP REMOVAL

Tips that have been glued to the nail plate can cause damage if removed improperly. Use a glue remover or acetone to remove tips.

1. **Complete nail tip application pre-service.** You will only need to add a buffer block to your manicuring table.

2. **Soak nails.** Place enough remover in a small glass bowl to cover nails. Soak nails for a few minutes.

3. **Slide off tip.** Use your orangewood stick to slide off softened tip. Be careful not to pry tip off because you can damage the nail bed and mantle. (Fig. 11.15)

4. **Buff nail.** Gently buff natural nail with fine block buffer to remove any glue residue. (Fig. 11.16)

5. **Condition cuticle and surrounding skin.** Condition cuticle and surrounding skin with cuticle oil and massage cream.

6. **Proceed to desired service.**

7. **Complete nail tip application post-service** if client is receiving no further service.

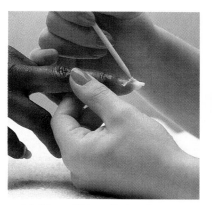

11.15 — Slide off tip; do not pry.

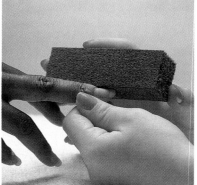

11.16 — Use fine buffer block to remove glue residue.

Review Questions

1. List the four supplies, in addition to your basic manicuring table, that you need for nail tip application.
2. Name the two types of nail tips.
3. What portion of the natural nail plate should be covered by a nail tip?
4. What type of tip application is considered a temporary service? Why?
5. Briefly describe the procedure for nail tip application.
6. Describe the proper maintenance of nail tips.
7. Describe the procedure for the removal of tips.

CHAPTER 12

Nail Wraps

LEARNING OBJECTIVES

After you have studied this chapter, you should be able to:
1. List four kinds of nail wraps.
2. Explain benefits of using silk, linen, fiberglass, and paper wraps.
3. Demonstrate the proper procedures and precautions to use in fabric wrap application.
4. Describe the maintenance of fabric wrap. Include a description of the two-week and four-week follow-up.
5. Explain how fabric wrap is used for crack repair.
6. Demonstrate the proper procedure and precautions for fabric wrap removal.
7. List the supplies used in paper wrap.
8. Demonstrate proper procedures for paper wrap application.
9. Define liquid nail wrap and describe its purpose.

Introduction

Nail wraps, sometimes called *overlays,* are nail-size pieces of cloth or paper that are bonded to the front of the nail plate with nail adhesive. They are used to repair or strengthen natural nails or nail tips. Wraps can be cut from a swatch of cloth or piece of paper to fit a client's nail size and shape, or they can be purchased pre-cut. Pre-cut overlays have an adhesive back and are attached only to the front of the nail.

Fabric wraps are made from silk, linen, or fiberglass. *Silk* is a thin natural material with a tight weave that becomes transparent when adhesive is applied. A silk wrap is strong, lightweight, and smooth when applied to the nail. *Linen* is a closely woven, heavy material. It is much thicker than silk or fiberglass. Because it is opaque, even after adhesive is applied, a colored polish must be used to cover it completely. Linen is a strong wrap and lasts a long time. *Fiberglass* is a very thin synthetic mesh with a loose weave. The loose weave makes it easy for adhesive to penetrate. It is especially strong and durable.

Paper wraps are made of very thin paper and dissolve in both acetone and non-acetone remover. For this reason, paper wraps are temporary and must be reapplied when polish is removed. Paper wraps are glued both on top of the nail and under the free edge.

Fabric Wraps

SUPPLIES

In addition to the materials on your basic manicuring table, you will need the following items: (Fig. 12.1)

Fabric. Small swatches of linen, silk, or fiberglass material that can be cut to fit a client's nail size and shape. You may also find pre-cut wraps with an adhesive backing.

Nail adhesive. Glue or bonding agent used to secure the nail tip or fabric to the natural nail. It usually comes in a tube with a pointed applicator tip called an *extender tip.*

Small scissors. Small and sharp for cutting fabric.

Nail block buffer.

Abrasive.

Adhesive dryer. Drop-on or spray that dries nail adhesive quickly.

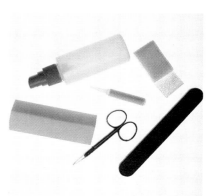

12.1 — Materials necessary for fabric wrap application

NAIL WRAP PRE-SERVICE

Use the following preparation for all nail wrap procedures.

1. Do the pre-service sanitation procedure. (This procedure is described on pages 29–30.)

2. Set up standard manicuring table. Add fabric, nail adhesive, small scissors, nail block buffer, abrasive, and adhesive dryer to your table.

3. Greet client and ask her to wash her hands in antibacterial soap. Dry hands and nails thoroughly with a fresh towel.

4. Do client consultation, using client record/health card to record the responses and your observations. Check for nail disorders. Decide if client's nails and hands are healthy enough for you to perform a service. If the client has a nail or skin disorder and should not receive a service, explain the reasons and refer the client to a doctor. If you proceed with the service, discuss your client's needs and wants.

NAIL WRAP PROCEDURE

During the procedure discuss with your client the products she will need to maintain the service between salon visits.

1. **Remove old polish.** Begin with the client's left hand, little finger. Saturate cotton with polish remover. If client is wearing artificial nails, use non-acetone remover to avoid damaging them. Hold saturated cotton on nail while you count to ten in your mind. Wipe the old polish off the nail with a stroking motion towards the free edge. If all polish is not removed, repeat this step until traces of polish are gone. It may be necessary to put cotton around the tip of an orangewood stick and use it to clean polish away from cuticle area. Repeat this procedure on each finger of both hands.

2. **Clean nails.** Dip nails in fingerbowls filled with warm water and antibacterial soap. Then use nail brush to clean nails over fingerbowl. Rinse nails briefly in clear water. DO NOT soak client's nails in water before you apply a nail wrap. When water is used to rinse the fingers, dip them very briefly in fingerbowl. Natural nails are porous and retain water. Water-soaked nails are a perfect breeding ground for mold and fungus under the nail wrap.

3. **Push back cuticle.** Use a cotton-tipped orangewood stick to gently push back cuticle. Use a light touch because the cuticle has not been soaked.

4. **Buff nail to remove shine.** Buff lightly over nail plate with medium/fine abrasive to remove the natural oil. Do not use a coarse file and be careful not to apply extreme pressure.

CHAPTER 12 NAIL WRAPS 143

5. **Apply nail antiseptic.** Use a cotton-tipped orangewood stick, cotton, or spray to apply nail antiseptic to nails. Begin with the little finger on the left hand and work toward the thumb. The antiseptic will remove the remaining natural oil and dehydrate the nail for better adhesion.

6. **Apply adhesive.** Apply adhesive to the entire surface of all ten nails. This prepares them to receive wraps. Let adhesive dry.

7. **Cut fabric.** Cut fabric to approximate width and shape of nail plate. (Fig. 12.2)

8. **Apply fabric adhesive.** Apply a drop of adhesive to center of nail. Keep adhesive off the cuticle because it will cause the wrap to lift or separate from the nail plate. (Fig. 12.3)

9. **Apply fabric.** Gently fit fabric over nail, 1/16 inch away from cuticle. Press to smooth. (Fig. 12.4)

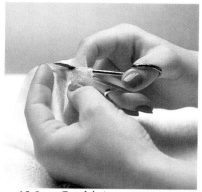

12.2 — Cut fabric.

PROCEDURAL TIP

▶ *Using a thick plastic sheet to press fabric onto nail will prevent the transfer of bacteria from you to your client.*

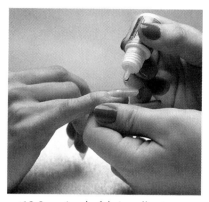

12.3 — Apply fabric adhesive.

10. **Trim fabric.** Use small scissors to trim fabric 1/16 inch away from sidewalls and free edge. Trimming fabric slightly smaller than nail plate prevents fabric from **lifting** or separating from the nail plate. (Fig. 12.5)

11. **Apply fabric adhesive.** Draw a thin coat of adhesive down the center of the nail using the extender tip to apply. Do not touch the cuticle. The adhesive will penetrate the fabric and stick to the nail surface. (Fig. 12.6)

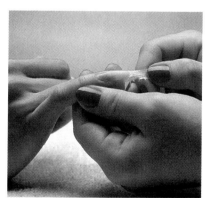

12.4 — Apply fabric.

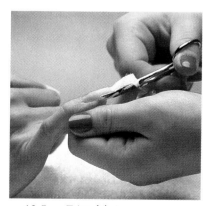

12.5 — Trim fabric.

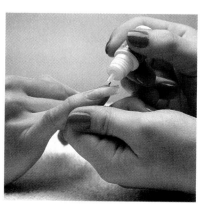

12.6 — Apply adhesive.

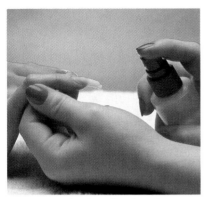

12.7 — Apply adhesive dryer.

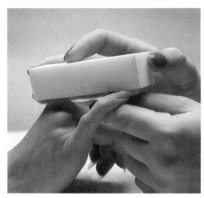

12.8 — Buff nails.

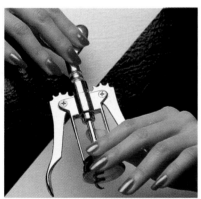

12.9 — Finished fabric wraps

12. **Apply adhesive dryer.** Spray or drop on adhesive dryer. Keep adhesive dryer off skin to prevent a heat sensation in your client's nail. If you are using spray adhesive dryer, hold the bottle at shoulder level and spray down on nail plate. (Fig. 12.7)
13. **Apply second coat of adhesive.** Apply and spread adhesive with extender tip. Seal free edge with adhesive by running the extender tip on the edge of the nail tip to prevent any lifting.
14. **Apply second coat of adhesive dryer.**
15. **Shape and refine nails.** Use medium/fine abrasive to shape and refine nails
16. **Buff nails.** Apply cuticle oil and buff to a high shine with block buffer. Brush block buffer over surface of nail to smooth out rough areas in fabric. Do not buff too much or too hard because you can wear through the wrap and weaken it. (Fig. 12.8)
17. **Apply hand lotion and massage hand and arm.**
18. **Remove traces of oil.** Use a small piece of cotton or a cotton-tipped orangewood stick to remove traces of oil from nail so alcohol or non-acetone polish will adhere.
19. **Apply polish.** (Fig. 12.9)

NAIL WRAP POST-SERVICE

Follow this post-service for all your nail wrap services.

1. **Make another appointment.** Schedule another appointment with your client to maintain the nail wrap she has just received or for another service.
2. **Sell retail products.** Suggest that your client buy products necessary to maintain her nails throughout the week. Polish, lotion, top coat, etc. are valuable maintenance tools for her to have.
3. **Clean up around your table.** Take the time to restore the basic set-up of your table. Cap adhesive and adhesive dryer to prevent evaporation.
4. **Clean extender tips.** To clean clogged extender tips, place them in a covered glass jar with acetone. Poke a clean toothpick through hole.
5. **Store fabric.** Store fabric in a sealable plastic bag to protect from bacteria.
6. **Discard used materials.** Place all used materials in the plastic bag at the side of the table. If the bag is full or contains used materials from artificial nail services, discard it in a closed pail.
7. **Sanitize table and implements.** Perform the complete pre-service sanitation procedure. Implements need to be sanitized 20 minutes before they can be used on the next client.

Wrap Up Profits with Nail Wraps

You can "wrap up" healthy profits and regular clients with nail wrap services. Nail wrapping began in the late '70s, when nail technicians used tea bags or paper to strengthen nails. As the service grew more popular, manufacturers introduced silk and linen wraps, and more recently, fiberglass wraps. Today linen wraps are the most popular, followed closely by silk. Fiberglass wraps are especially popular with clients who want to strengthen their natural nails while they grow out.

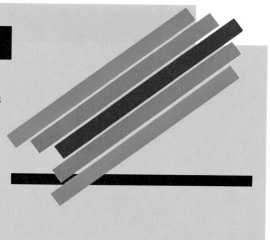

Fabric Wrap Maintenance, Removal, and Repairs

Fabric wraps need regular maintenance to keep them looking fresh. In this section you will learn how to maintain fabric wraps after two weeks and after four weeks. You will also learn how to remove fabric wraps and how to use fabric wraps for crack repair.

FABRIC WRAP MAINTENANCE

Fabric wraps are maintained with glue "fills" after two weeks and with glue and fabric "fills" after four weeks.

Two-Week Maintenance

After two weeks use the following procedure to maintain fabric wraps. You will need to add nail adhesive, a nail block buffer, and adhesive dryer to your standard table set-up.

1. **Complete nail wrap pre-service.**
2. **Remove old polish.** Use a non-acetone polish remover to avoid damaging wraps.
3. **Clean nails.**
4. **Push back cuticle.**
5. **Buff nail to remove shine.** Make sure the line between the new growth and the existing wrap is smooth.
6. **Apply nail antiseptic.**
7. **Apply adhesive to new nail growth area.** Apply a small drop of adhesive to new nail growth. Spread with extender tip, taking care not to touch skin.
8. **Apply adhesive dryer.**

9. **Apply adhesive to entire nail.** Apply a second coat of adhesive to entire nail to strengthen and reseal wrap.
10. **Apply adhesive dryer.**
11. **Shape and refine nail.** Use medium/fine abrasive over surface of nail to remove any peaks and imperfections.
12. **Buff nails.** Apply cuticle oil and buff to a high shine with block buffer.
13. **Apply hand lotion and massage hand and arm.**
14. **Remove traces of oil.** Use a small piece of cotton or a cotton-tipped orangewood stick to remove traces of oil from nail so polish will adhere.
15. **Apply polish.**
16. **Complete nail wrap post-service.**

Four-Week Maintenance

After four weeks use the following maintenance procedure to apply fabric and adhesive to new growth. You will need nail adhesive, a nail block buffer, fabric, small scissors, and adhesive dryer in addition to your standard table set-up.

1. **Complete nail wrap pre-service.**
2. **Remove old polish.** Use a non-acetone polish remover to avoid damaging wraps.
3. **Clean nails.** Use nail brush and antibacterial soap to gently clean nails.
4. **Push back cuticle.**
5. **Buff nail to remove shine.** Lightly buff over nail plates to remove natural oil and to remove any small pieces of fabric that may have lifted. Buff nail until smooth, without scratching natural nail plate. Totally refine nail until there is no line of demarcation between new growth and fabric wrap.
6. **Apply nail antiseptic.**
7. **Cut fabric.** Cut a piece of fabric large enough to cover the new growth area above the old wrap.
8. **Apply fabric.** Gently fit fabric over new growth area and smooth. (Fig. 12.10)
9. **Trim fabric.** Trim fabric 1/16 inch away from cuticle and sides of nail. Allow new fabric to slightly overlap existing fabric.
10. **Apply adhesive to regrowth area.** Apply a small drop of adhesive to fabric in new growth area. Spread throughout new growth area with the extender tip. Be careful to avoid cuticle or skin. (Fig. 12.11)
11. **Apply adhesive dryer.**
12. **Apply adhesive.** Apply a second coat of adhesive to regrowth area.
13. **Apply second coat of adhesive dryer.**

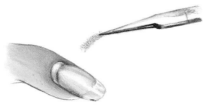

12.10 — Apply fabric to regrowth area.

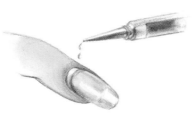

12.11 — Apply adhesive to regrowth area.

14. **Apply adhesive to entire nail.** Apply a thin coat of adhesive to entire nail to strengthen and seal wrap.

15. **Apply adhesive dryer.**

16. **Shape and refine nail.** Use medium/fine abrasive over surface of nail to remove any peaks and imperfections. Carefully stay away from cuticle so you do not cut and damage skin.

17. **Buff nails.** Apply cuticle oil and buff to a high shine with block buffer.

18. **Apply hand lotion and massage hand and arm.**

19. **Remove traces of oil.** Use a small piece of cotton or a cotton-tipped orangewood stick and acetone to remove traces of oil from nail so polish will adhere.

20. **Apply polish.**

21. **Complete nail wrap post-service.**

REPAIRS WITH FABRIC WRAPS

Small pieces of fabric can be used to strengthen a weak point in the nail or repair a break in the nail. A *stress strip* is a strip of fabric cut to 1/8 inch. The strip is applied to the weak point of the nail, using the four-week maintenance procedure. A *repair patch* is a piece of fabric that is cut so it completely covers the crack or break in the nail. Use the four-week fabric wrap maintenance procedure to apply your repair patch.

FABRIC WRAP REMOVAL

Be careful not to damage the nail plate when removing fabric wraps.

1. **Complete nail wrap pre-service.**

2. **Soak nails.** Put enough acetone in a small glass bowl to cover the nails. Immerse client's nails in bowl and soak for a few minutes.

3. **Slide off softened wraps.** Use an orangewood stick to slide softened wraps away from nail.

4. **Buff nails.** Gently buff natural nails with fine block buffer to remove the glue residue.

5. **Condition cuticles.** Condition cuticles and surrounding skin with cuticle oil and lotion.

Paper Wraps

Paper wraps are applied as a temporary method of strengthening the nail. Mending tissue, a thin paper, is applied over the nail plate to add strength to a nail just as a fabric does. Paper wraps are temporary because they are applied with mending liquid, which dissolves in polish remover. Therefore, the wrap is removed each time the polish is removed. Paper wraps provide added strength for a short period of time. These wraps are not recommended for extra long nails because they do not provide the strength that long nails require.

SUPPLIES

Mending tissue. A lightweight thin tissue paper.

Mending liquid. A heavy liquid adhesive that dissolves in polish remover. It is applied with a brush.

Ridge filler.

Paper Wrap Application Procedure

1. **Complete nail wrap pre-service.** Add mending liquid, mending tissue, and ridge filler to your table.
2. **Remove old polish.**
3. **Clean nails.** Use nail brush and antibacterial soap to gently scrub nails.
4. **Push back cuticle.**
5. **Buff nails to remove shine.** Use medium/fine abrasive to remove shine from nails.
6. **Apply nail antiseptic.** Use cotton-tipped orangewood stick, cotton, or spray to apply nail antiseptic to all nails.
7. **Tear mending tissue.** Tear tissue to fit the shape of the nail, making sure it is feathered at the edges. The tissue should be long enough to tuck under the free edge. (Fig. 12.12)
8. **Apply mending liquid to tissue.** Saturate each piece of tissue with mending liquid.
9. **Apply tissue.** Place wrap over the nail using two fingers. (Fig. 12.13)

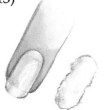

12.12 — Tear mending tissue.

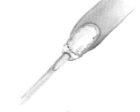

12.13 — Apply tissue.

CHAPTER 12 NAIL WRAPS 149

10. **Smooth the wrap.** Use a steel pusher or orangewood stick to push tissue toward the free edge and sidewalls. Dip pusher into polish remover repeatedly and pat tissue until it is smooth.
11. **Trim excess tissue.** Trim tissue 1/16 inch from the sidewalls. Leave enough tissue at the end to wrap under free edge. (Fig. 12.14)
12. **Apply mending liquid under free edge.** Turn the finger over and apply mending liquid under free edge.
13. **Smooth wrap.** Use pusher to smooth wrap under free edge. (Fig. 12.15)

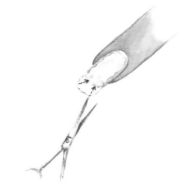

12.14 — Cut slits into tissue.

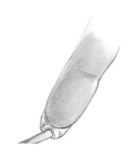

12.15 — Smooth wrap under free edge.

14. **Refine nail.** Gently smooth top of the wrap with the fine side of an emery board. This removes any minute particles that may cause bubbling.
15. **Apply mending liquid.** Apply two or three coats of mending liquid to the top and underside of the free edge of the nail.
16. **Apply ridge filler.** Apply a thin coat of ridge filler to top of nails to smooth surface. Allow filler to dry completely before applying polish.
17. **Apply polish.**
18. **Complete nail wrap post-service.** (Fig. 12.16)

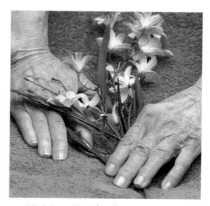

12.16 — Finished paper wrap.

Liquid Nail Wrap

Liquid nail wrap is a polish made up of tiny fibers designed to strengthen and preserve the natural nail as it grows. It is brushed on the nail in several directions to create a network that, once hardened, protects the nail. It is similar to nail hardener, but thicker because it contains more fiber.

Review Questions

1. List four kinds of nail wraps.
2. Explain the benefits of using silk, linen, fiberglass, and paper wraps.
3. Describe the procedure for fabric wrap application.
4. Explain how a fabric wrap is used as a crack repair.
5. Describe how to remove fabric wraps and what to avoid.
6. Describe the purpose of paper wraps and explain why they are not recommended for very long nails.
7. List the materials used for paper wraps.
8. Outline the procedures used in paper wraps.
9. Define liquid nail wrap and describe its purpose.

CHAPTER 13

Acrylic Nails

LEARNING OBJECTIVES

After you have studied this chapter, you should be able to:
1. Identify the supplies needed for acrylic nail application.
2. Explain the chemistry of acrylic nails.
3. Demonstrate the proper procedure and precautions for the application of acrylic nails over forms.
4. Describe the safety precautions for applying primer.
5. Demonstrate the proper procedure and precautions for the application of acrylic nails over tips.
6. Demonstrate the proper procedure and precautions for acrylic nail application over bitten nails.
7. Describe two basic types of maintenance for acrylic nails.
8. Describe the proper procedure for removing acrylics.
9. Explain how the application of odorless acrylics differs from the application of traditional acrylics.

Introduction

Acrylic (a-**KRYL**-yk), or sculptured nails are made by combining a liquid acrylic product with a powdered acrylic product. The two products form a soft ball that can easily be molded into a nail shape. After it is applied, the soft acrylic hardens into a strong artificial nail. Acrylic nails can be applied to natural nails, nail tips, or nail forms to strengthen or extend the nail. They can also be used to repair weak, bitten, and torn nails. The nail technician builds the nail to conform to the shape of the client's fingers and hands for natural-looking, durable nails.

The basic chemistry of acrylic nails is simple. There are three basic ingredients in the acrylic nail process. A *monomer* (**MON**-oh-mehr) is something made up of many small molecules that are not attached to one another. Liquid acrylic is a type of monomer. A *polymer* (**POL**-i-mehr) is made up of molecules that are attached in long chains and usually form something hard. Finished acrylic nails are polymers. A *catalyst* (**CAT**-a-lyst) is an ingredient that speeds up the hardening process. The hardening process is also referred to as **curing**. The powdered acrylic used is a combination of ground-up polymer and a catalyst. The process of forming the nail is called *polymerization* (pol-i-mehr-i-**ZAY**-shun).

Acrylic Nails over Forms

There are two acrylic nail methods—one-color and two-color. The one-color method uses a single color of acrylic powder (clear, natural, or pink) for the entire nail and produces a nail that is usually worn with polish. The two-color method uses white acrylic powder for the free edge and clear, natural, or pink powder for the nail bed. It produces a nail that looks as if it has a French manicure and needs no polish.

SUPPLIES FOR ACRYLIC NAILS

In addition to the supplies in your basic manicuring set-up, you will need the following items: (Fig. 13.1)

Acrylic liquid. Combined with the acrylic powder to form the sculptured nail. Also referred to as a monomer.

Acrylic powder. White, clear, natural, and pink powder is available. The color(s) you choose will depend on the acrylic nail method you are using.

Primer. Applied to the nail so that the acrylic product will adhere to the natural nail. Primer can be non-etching or etching. *Non-etching primer* is easier to use safely but may not be as effective as etching primer. *Etching primers* chemically dissolve nooks and

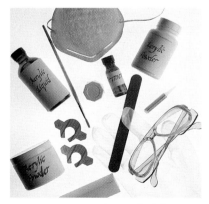

13.1 — Materials needed for application of acrylic nails.

crannies into the natural nail to help the acrylic to hold on to the nail plate. Primers are very effective but can cause serious, sometimes irreversible, damage to skin and eyes. Never use primer without plastic gloves and safety glasses.

Abrasive.

Small containers for liquid and powdered acrylic.

Nail forms. Can be disposable or reusable. Disposable forms have an adhesive backing that holds the form in place. Resuable forms are made of aluminum, Teflon, or plastic and have no adhesive backing.

Sable brush. Used to apply and shape the soft balls of acrylic on the nail.

Safety glasses.

Plastic gloves.

Safety mask. (optional)

ACRYLIC NAIL PRE-SERVICE

1. Complete Pre-Service Sanitation Procedure. (This procedure is described on pages 29–30.)
2. Set up your standard manicuring table. Add the acrylic materials to your table.
3. Greet client and ask her to wash hands with antibacterial soap. Be sure to dry hands thoroughly with a fresh towel.
4. Do client consultation, using client health/record card to record responses and observations. Check for nail disorders and decide if it is safe and appropriate to perform a service on this client. If the client should not receive a service, explain your reasons and refer her to a doctor.

ACRYLIC NAIL PROCEDURE

1. **Remove polish.** Begin with your client's left hand, little finger, and work toward the thumb. Then repeat on the right hand.
2. **Clean nails.** Ask client to dip nails in fingerbowl filled with antibacterial soap. Then use nail brush to clean nails over fingerbowl. Rinse nails briefly in clear water. DO NOT soak client's nails in water before you apply an acrylic nail. When water is used to rinse the fingers, dip them very briefly in fingerbowl. Natural nails are porous and retain water. Water-soaked nails are a perfect breeding ground for bacteria that may produce mold and fungus under the acrylic nail. (Fig. 13.2)
3. **Push back cuticle.** Use a cotton-tipped orangewood stick to gently push back cuticle.
4. **Buff nail to remove shine.** Buff lightly over nail plate with medium/fine abrasive to remove the natural oil. Brush off filings. (Fig. 13.3)

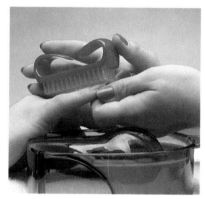

13.2 — Clean nails.

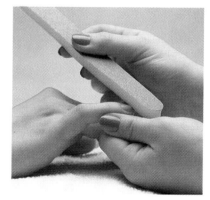

13.3 — Buff nail to remove shine.

154 PART IV THE ART OF NAIL TECHNOLOGY

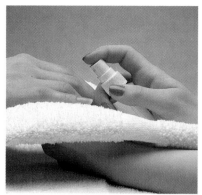

13.4 — Apply nail antiseptic.

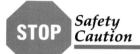 **Safety Caution**

Be very careful not to allow primer to touch your client's skin or your own. If you accidently spill primer on your clothing, remove the soiled garment immediately.

5. **Apply nail antiseptic.** Apply nail antiseptic to nails with cotton-tipped orangewood stick, cotton, or spray. Begin with the little finger on the left hand and work toward the thumb. (Fig. 13.4)

6. **Position nail form.** Position nail form on nail. If you are using disposable forms, peel a nail form from its paper backing and, using the thumb and index finger of each of your hands, bend the form into an arch to fit the client's natural nail shape. Slide the form onto your client's finger and press adhesive backing to sides of the finger. Check to see that the form is snug under the free edge and level with the natural nail.

   If you are using reusable forms, slide the form onto the client's finger, making sure the free edge is over the form and that it fits snugly. Be careful not to cut into the part of the skin under the free edge. Tighten the form around the finger by squeezing lightly. (Fig. 13.5)

7. **Apply primer.** Put on plastic gloves and a pair of safety glasses. Offer a pair of safety glasses to your client. Apply a dot of primer on nail with a cotton-tipped orangewood stick. The primer prepares the nail surface for bonding with the acrylic material. Primer should be applied very sparingly. Allow primer to dry on nail to a chalky white. (Figs. 13.6, 13.7)

8. **Prepare acrylic liquid and powder.** Pour acrylic liquid and acrylic powder into separate small containers. If you are using the two-color method, you will need three small containers—one for the white tip powder, one for the clear, natural, or pink powder, and one for the acrylic liquid. (Throughout this chapter, pink and white acrylic powders are used for the two-color method. Your client may select the one-color method or she may pick clear or natural powder instead of pink.)

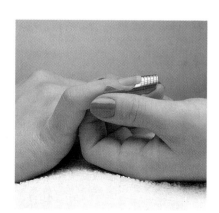

13.5 — Position nail form.

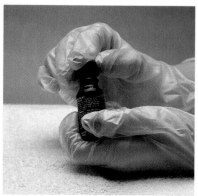

13.6 — Always use plastic gloves when applying primer.

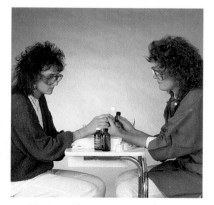

13.7 — Always wear safety glasses when apply primer.

9. **Dip brush into acrylic liquid.** Dip brush fully into the liquid and wipe on the edge of the container to remove the excess. (Fig. 13.8)

10. **Form acrylic ball.** Dip the tip of the same brush into the white acrylic powder and rotate slightly. You will pick up a ball of acrylic product of medium-dry consistency that is large enough for shaping the entire free edge extension. (Fig. 13.9)

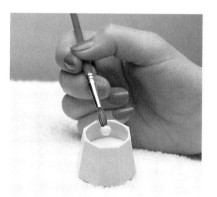

13.8 — Dip brush into acrylic liquid.

PROCEDURAL TIP

▶ *Do not touch primed area of the nail with wet brush until you apply acrylic on the area. The acrylic will lift if the area has been touched with the wet brush.*

11. **Place ball of acrylic.** Place acrylic ball on the nail form at the point where the free edge joins the nail form. (Figs. 13.10, 13.11)

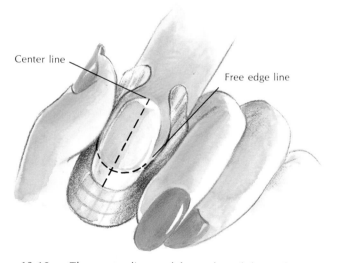

13.10 — The center line and free edge of the nail

13.9 — Form ball of acrylic.

12. **Shape free edge.** Use the middle portion of your sable brush to dab and press the acrylic to shape an extension. Do not "paint" the acrylic onto the nail. Dabbing and pressing the acrylic is more accurate than "painting" and produces a more natural-looking nail. Keep sidewall lines parallel and shape acrylic continuously along free edge line. If you are using the

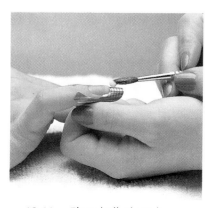

13.11 — Place ball of acrylic on nail form.

two-color acrylic method, make sure you follow the natural free edge line with the white powder to produce the French manicure look. (Figs. 13.12, 13.13)

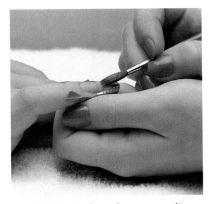

13.12 — Dab and press acrylic with the middle portion of brush.

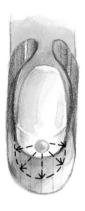

13.13 — Shape free edge.

13. **Place second ball of acrylic.** Pick up a second ball of acrylic of medium consistency and place it on natural nail next to the free edge line in center of nail. (Fig. 13.14)
14. **Shape second ball of acrylic.** Dab and press product to sidewalls, making sure the product is very thin around all edges. If you are using a two-color acrylic product, use the pink powder in this step. (Fig. 13.15)
15. **Apply acrylic beads.** Pick up small wet beads of pink acrylic powder on your brush and place at cuticle area. Use the moisture in the brush to smooth these beads over entire nail plate. Glide brush over nail to smooth out imperfections. Acrylic application near cuticle, sidewall, and free edge should be extremely thin for a natural-looking nail. (Fig. 13.16)

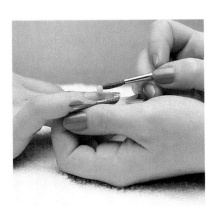

13.14 — Place ball on natural nail.

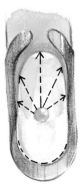

13.15 — Shape second ball of acrylic.

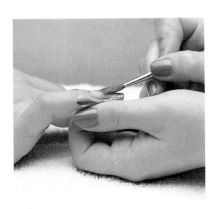

13.16 — Apply acrylic beads.

PROCEDURAL TIP

▶ Acrylic applied too thickly near cuticle can cause acrylic nail to lift.

16. **Apply acrylic to remaining nails.** Repeat steps 5–14 on remaining nails.

17. **Remove forms.** When nails are thoroughly dry, loosen forms and slide them off. Nails are dry when they make a clicking sound when lightly tapped. (Fig. 13.17)

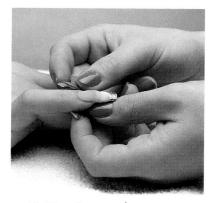

13.17 — Remove forms.

18. **Shape nails.** Use coarse/medium abrasive to shape free edge and to remove imperfections. Glide abrasive over each nail with long sweeping strokes to further shape and perfect nail surface. Make nails thinner toward cuticles, free edge, and sidewalls.

19. **Buff nails.** Buff nails with block buffer until entire surface is smooth.

20. **Apply cuticle oil.** Use a cotton-tipped orangewood stick to apply cuticle oil to cuticles, surrounding skin, and nails. (Fig. 13.18)

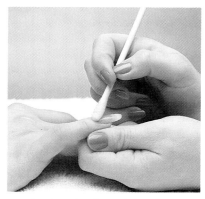

13.18 — Apply cuticle oil.

21. **Apply hand cream and massage hand and arm.**

22. **Clean nails.** Ask client to dip nails in fingerbowl filled with antibacterial soap. Then use nail brush to clean nails over fingerbowl. Rinse with water. Dry thoroughly. If your client selected the two-color method, her acrylic nails are finished. (Fig. 13.19)

23. **Apply polish.** If your client selected one-color acrylic nails, apply the polish she has chosen.

ACRYLIC POST-SERVICE

1. **Make another appointment.** Schedule another appointment with your client for maintaining her acrylic nails. A fill-in will be necessary in two or three weeks, depending on how quickly the nails grow. Encourage your client to return for a water manicure between acrylic maintenance appointments if her acrylic nails are polished.

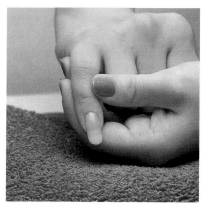

13.19 — Finished acrylic nail

2. **Sell retail products.** Suggest that your client buy products necessary to maintain her acrylic nails between appointments. Polish, lotion, and top coat may be helpful.

3. **Clean up around your table.** Take the time to restore the basic set-up of your table. Be sure that all your acrylic product bottles are closed tightly.

4. **Clean brush.** Clean brush in acetone or in manufacturer's cleaner. Never pull out bristles of brush because you will loosen the remaining bristles. Clip one stray hair if necessary but never trim bristles because you will ruin the accuracy of the brush.

5. **Store acrylic products.** Store acrylic powders in covered containers. Store all primers and acrylic liquids in a cool, dark area. Do not store products near heat.

6. **Discard used materials.** Never save used primer or liquid that has been removed from original bottle. Use on one client only, then pour leftover liquid into plastic bag. Place all used materials in the plastic bag at the side of the table. After all used materials have been placed in the bag, discard it in a closed pail. Since acrylic products can produce harmful vapors, it is important to remove items soiled with acrylic product from your manicuring station after each client.

7. **Sanitize table and implements.** Perform the complete pre-service sanitation procedure. Implements must be sanitized for 20 minutes before they can be used on another client. Reusable forms must be sanitized for at least 20 minutes in an approved disinfectant since they will be used again.

Acrylic Nails over Tips or Natural Nails

PROCEDURE

1. **Complete acrylic nail pre-service.** This procedure is described on page 153.

2. **Remove polish.** Begin with your client's left hand, little finger, and work toward the thumb. Then repeat on the right hand.

3. **Clean nails.** Ask client to dip nails in fingerbowl filled with anitbacterial soap. Then use nail brush to clean nails over fingerbowl. Rinse nails briefly in clear water.

4. **Push back cuticle.** Use an orangewood stick to gently push back cuticle.

5. **Buff nail to remove shine.** Buff lightly over nail plate with medium/fine abrasive to remove the natural oil. Brush off filings.

6. **Apply nail antiseptic.** Apply nail antiseptic to nails with cotton-tipped orangewood stick, cotton, or spray. Begin with the little finger on the left hand and work toward the thumb.

7. **Apply tips.** Apply tips if your client desires them, using the technique described in Chapter 11.

8. **Apply primer.** Put on plastic gloves and a pair of safety glasses. Offer a pair of safety glasses to your client. Apply a dot of primer on nail and nail tip (if instructed by tip manufacturer) with a cotton-tipped orangewood stick. Allow primer to dry to chalky white color before applying acrylic.

9. **Prepare acrylic liquid and powder.** Pour acrylic liquid and acrylic powder into separate small containers. If you are using the two-color system, you will need three small containers—one for the white tip powder, one for the pink powder, and one for the acrylic liquid.

10. **Dip brush into liquid.** Dip brush fully into the liquid and wipe on the edge of the container to remove the excess.

11. **Form acrylic ball.** Dip the tip of the same brush into the white acrylic powder and rotate slightly. You will pick up a medium/dry ball of acrylic product that is large enough to shape the entire free edge.

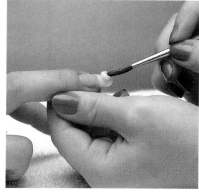
13.20 — Place ball of acrylic on free edge.

12. **Place ball of acrylic on free edge.** Place acrylic ball on the free edge of tip or natural nail. (Fig. 13.20)

13. **Shape free edge.** Use the middle portion of your sable brush to dab and press the acrylic to shape the free edge. Keep sidewall lines parallel. Do not ''paint'' acrylic onto nail. If you are using the two-color acrylic method, make sure you follow the natural free edge line with the white powder to produce a French manicure look.

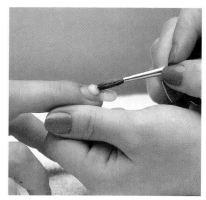
13.21 — Place second ball of acrylic on nail bed.

14. **Place second ball of acrylic.** Pick up a second ball of acrylic of medium consistency and place it on the nail bed next to the free edge line in center of nail. (Fig. 13.21)

15. **Shape second ball of acrylic.** Dab and press product to sidewalls and cuticle, making sure the product is very thin around all edges. If you are using a two-color acrylic product, use the pink powder in this step.

16. **Apply acrylic beads.** Pick up small wet beads of acrylic powder on your brush and place at cuticle area. Use the moisture in the brush to smooth these beads over entire nail. Glide brush over nail to smooth out imperfections. Keep acrylic application near cuticle, sidewall, and free edge extremely thin for the most natural-looking nail. For the two-color method use pink powder to form acrylic beads. (Fig. 13.22)

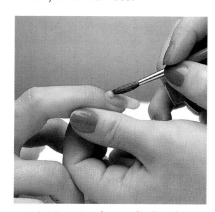
13.22 — Apply acrylic beads.

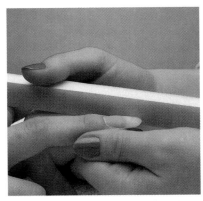

13.23 — Shape and refine nail.

17. **Shape and refine nail.** Use coarse abrasive to shape free edge and to remove imperfections. Then refine with medium/fine abrasive. (Fig. 13.23)
18. **Buff nails.** Buff nail with block buffer until entire surface is smooth. (Fig. 13.24)
19. **Apply cuticle oil.** Rub cuticle oil into cuticles surrounding skin and nail surface.
20. **Apply hand cream and massage hand and arm.**
21. **Clean nails.** Ask client to dip nails in fingerbowl filled with antibacterial soap. Then use nail brush to clean nails over fingerbowl. Rinse with water. Dry thoroughly. Two-color acrylic nails are now finished. (Fig. 13.25)
22. **Apply polish.** Polish one-color acrylic nails.
23. **Complete acrylic post-service procedure.**

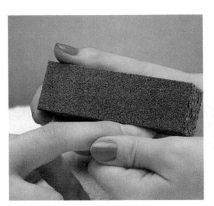

13.24 — Buff nails until smooth.

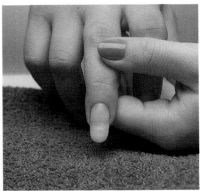

13.25 — Finished acrylic nail over tip.

Acrylic Nail Application over Bitten Nails

PROCEDURE

The procedure for applying acrylic nails over bitten nails is similar to the application of acrylic nails over forms. However, you must create a portion of the nail plate before applying the nail form.

1. **Complete acrylic application pre-service.**
2. **Remove polish.** Begin with your client's left hand, little finger, and work toward the thumb. Then repeat on the right hand.
3. **Clean nails.** Ask client to dip nails in fingerbowl filled with antibacterial soap. Then use nail brush to clean nails over fingerbowl. Rinse nails briefly in clear water.
4. **Push back cuticle.** Use an orangewood stick to gently push back cuticle.

5. **Buff nail to remove shine.** Buff lightly over nail plate with medium/fine abrasive to remove the natural oil. Brush off filings.
6. **Apply nail antiseptic.** Apply nail antiseptic to nails with cotton-tipped orangewood, cotton, or spray. Begin with the little finger on the left hand and work toward the thumb.
7. **Apply primer.** Put on plastic gloves and a pair of safety glasses. Offer a pair of safety glasses to your client. Apply a dot of primer on nail plate with a cotton-tipped orangewood stick. Primer is meant for the nail plate only. People with bitten nails often have rough cuticles and damaged surrounding skin. Be very careful to avoid touching any of the client's skin with primer.
8. **Prepare acrylic liquid and powder.** Pour acrylic liquid and acrylic powder into separate small containers.
9. **Form acrylic ball.** Pick up a small ball of acrylic product of medium/dry consistency. Use white for the two-color method.
10. **Place ball of acrylic on skin.** Apply a small ball of acrylic product on skin near bitten nail. (Fig. 13.26)
11. **Create nail plate.** Use the middle of your brush to dab and press to shape a nail plate or a base for the form on which the acrylic nail will be built. Do not place acrylic product beyond the sidewall line. (Fig. 13.27)
12. **Pull skin away.** Allow the acrylic to dry completely. You should be able to hear a click when you tap it with a brush. Then gently pull the client's skin away at the free edge line. You will now have a free edge that is large enough to support a nail form. (Fig. 13.28)

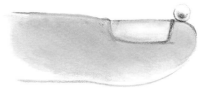

13.26 — Place ball of acrylic on skin.

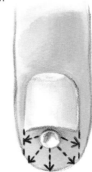

13.27 — Create nail plate.

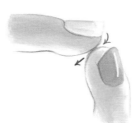

13.28 — Pull skin away.

13. **Position nail form.** Position nail form under newly created free edge.
14. **Place ball of acrylic.** Pick up ball of acrylic of medium consistency and place it on the nail form where the nail meets the nail form.
15. **Shape free edge.** Use the middle of your brush to dab and press the acrylic to shape an extension. Make free edge extend only slightly beyond fingertip because people with bitten nails are not used to having long nails.

16. **Place second ball of acrylic.** Pick up a second ball of acrylic of medium consistency and place it next to the free edge line in center of nail. If you are using the two-color method, use pink powder.
17. **Shape second ball of acrylic.** Dab and press product to sidewalls and cuticle area, making sure the product is very thin around all edges.
18. **Apply acrylic beads.** Pick up small wet beads of acrylic powder and place at cuticle area. Use the moisture in the brush to smooth these beads over cuticle and over entire nail plate. If you are using a two-color product use pink powder.
19. **Remove forms.** When nails are thoroughly dry, loosen forms and slide them off. Nails are dry when they make a clicking sound when lightly tapped.
20. **Shape nail.** Use coarse/medium abrasive to shape free edge and to remove imperfections.
21. **Buff nail.** Buff nail with block buffer until entire surface is smooth.
22. **Apply cuticle oil.** Rub cuticle oil into surrounding skin and nail surface.
23. **Apply hand cream and massage hand and arm.**
24. **Clean nails.** Ask client to dip nails in fingerbowl filled with antibacterial soap. Then use nail brush to clean nails over fingerbowl. Rinse with water. Dry thoroughly. Your two-color acrylic nails are finished.
25. **Apply polish.** Polish one-color acrylic nails.
26. **Complete acrylic application post-service.**

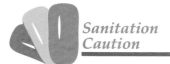

Sanitation Caution

Check primer for clarity on a regular basis to make sure it is not contaminated with bacteria. If bacteria are present, the primer will appear grainy and cloudy.

Acrylic Nail Maintenance and Removal

Regular maintenance helps prevent acrylic nails from lifting or cracking. When acrylic nails lift, crack, or grow out with no maintenance, moisture and dirt can become trapped under the acrylic nail and fungus can begin to grow.

ACRYLIC MAINTENANCE

There are two basic types of maintenance for acrylic nails—fill-in and crack repair.

Fill-In

Fill-in is the addition of acrylic to the new growth area of the nails. Acrylic nails should be filled in every two to three weeks, depending on how fast the nail grows. Without a fill-in, the nail will begin to look unnatural and uneven as it grows longer. The new growth area near the cuticle will be noticeably lower than the rest of the nail.

Use the following procedure for fill-ins.

1. **Complete acrylic application pre-service.**

2. **Remove old polish.**

3. **Smooth ledge between new growth and acrylic nail.** Use a medium/fine abrasive to smooth the ledge of acrylic in the new growth area so that it blends into nail bed. (Fig. 13.29)

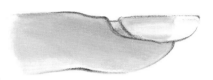

13.29 — New growth area that needs fill-in acrylic maintenance.

4. **Refine entire nail.** Hold abrasive flat and glide it over entire nail to reshape and refine nail and thin out free edge.

5. **Buff Nail.** Use buffer block to buff acrylic and blend it into new growth area.

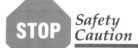

Safety Caution

6. **Blend acrylic that has lifted.** Use a file to smooth out any acrylic that might have lifted.

7. **Clean nail.** Use fingerbowl filled with warm water and antibacterial soap and a nail brush to gently wash nails. Do not soak nails.

8. **Push back cuticle.** Use a cotton-tipped orangewood stick to gently push back cuticle.

Do not use a nipper to clip away loose acrylic. Nipping may perpetuate the lifting problem and can damage the nail plate. If lifting is excessive, soak off acrylic and start fresh with a new nail application.

9. **Buff nail to remove shine.** Buff lightly over nail plate with medium/fine abrasive to remove the natural oil. Brush off filings.

10. **Apply nail antiseptic.** Apply nail antiseptic to nails with cotton-tipped orangewood stick, cotton, or spray.

11. **Apply primer.** Put on plastic gloves and a pair of safety glasses. Offer a pair of safety glasses to your client. Apply a dot of primer to the newly grown natural nail.

12. **Prepare acrylic liquid and powder.** Pour acrylic liquid and acrylic powder into separate small containers.

13. **Place balls of acrylic.** Pick up one or more small balls of acrylic and place them on the new growth area. Be sure to use pink acrylic if you are using a two-color method.

14. **Shape balls of acrylic.** Use middle of brush to dab and press the acrylic until it blends into the existing sculptured nail.

15. **Place balls of acrylic.** Pick up one or more small wet balls of acrylic and place them at the base of the nail bed towards the cuticle.

16. **Shape beads of acrylic.** Use the moisture in the brush to smooth these beads over entire nail plate. Glide brush over nail to smooth out imperfections. Acrylic application near cuticle, sidewall, and free edge should be extremely thin for a natural-looking nail. If you are using a two-color acrylic product, use the pink powder in this step.

17. **Shape nails.** Allow nails to dry thoroughly. Nails are dry when they make a clicking sound when lightly tapped. Use a coarse/medium grit abrasive to shape free edge and remove any imperfections. Use medium/fine abrasive to glide over nail with long sweeping strokes to further shape and perfect nail surface. Taper nail shape towards cuticle, nail tip, and sidewalls, making it thin at all edges. (After four or five weeks of growth and two fill-ins, the white acrylic free edge created with the two-color method grows beyond the natural free edge. At this time, your client may want to start wearing polish, and she may want you to file back the white free edge to create a one-color nail.)

18. **Buff nail.** Smooth entire surface of nail using block buffer until it is smooth.

19. **Apply cuticle oil.** Rub cuticle oil into surrounding skin, cuticle, and nail surface using a cotton-tipped orangewood stick.

20. **Apply hand cream and massage hand and arm.**

21. **Clean nails.**

22. **Apply polish.**

23. **Complete acrylic application post-service.**

Crack Repair

Acrylic crack repair is the addition of extra acrylic to fill the crack in an acrylic nail and reinforce the rest of the nail.

Use the following procedure for crack repairs.

1. **Complete acrylic application pre-service.**

2. **Remove old polish.**

3. **File cracked acrylic.** File a "V" shape into the crack or file flush to remove crack.

4. **Clean nails.** Ask client to dip nails in fingerbowl filled with warm water and antibacterial soap. Then use nail brush to clean nails over fingerbowl. Rinse nails briefly in clear water. Dry nails thoroughly.

5. **Apply nail antiseptic.** Apply nail antiseptic to nails using cotton-tipped orangewood stick, cotton, or spray.

6. **Apply primer.** If natural nail plate is exposed, put on plastic gloves and a pair of safety glasses and apply a dot of primer to the area.

CHAPTER 13 ACRYLIC NAILS

7. **Apply nail form.** If the crack is large, apply a nail form for added support.
8. **Prepare acrylic liquid and powder.** Pour acrylic liquid and acrylic powder into separate small containers.
9. **Place balls of acrylic.** Pick up one or more small beads of acrylic and apply them to the cracked area. If you are using the two-color system, be sure to use the correct color acrylic.
10. **Shape balls of acrylic.** Dab and press the acrylic to fill crack. Be careful not to let acrylic seep under form or under existing nail.
11. **Place additional balls of acrylic.** Apply additional acrylic, if needed, to fill in crack or reinforce the rest of the nail. Shape acrylic and allow it to dry thoroughly.
12. **Remove form (if used).**
13. **Reshape nail.**
14. **Buff until smooth.**
15. **Clean nails.**
16. **Apply cuticle oil.**
17. **Apply hand cream and massage hand and arm.**
18. **Clean nails.**
19. **Apply polish.**
20. **Complete acrylic application post-service.**

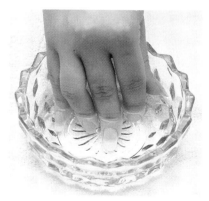

13.30 — Soak fingertips in acetone.

ACRYLIC REMOVAL

1. **Fill bowl with acetone.** Fill glass bowl with enough acetone to cover client's fingertips.
2. **Soak fingertips.** Soak client's fingertips for 15 minutes or as long as needed to remove acrylic product. Refer to your manufacturer's directions for acrylic removal. (Fig. 13.30)
3. **Remove acrylic with orangewood stick.** Use orangewood stick and gently push off softened acrylic nail. Repeat until all acrylic has been removed. Do not pry off acrylic with nippers, as this will damage natural nail plate. (Fig. 13.31)
4. **Buff nails.** Gently buff natural nail with fine block buffer to remove the acrylic residue.
5. **Condition cuticle.** Condition cuticle and surrounding skin with cuticle oil and hand lotion.

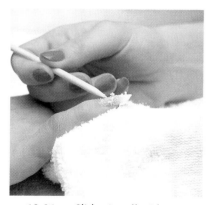

13.31 — Slide tip off with orangewood stick.

Odorless Acrylics

Odorless acrylics are acrylic products that do not smell as strongly as traditional acrylic products. They are useful if you or your clients are bothered by the odor of acrylic liquid. Although they are not completely odorless, they have less odor and are wetter than the traditional acrylic product.

Most odorless acrylics are self-leveling. As the product sets, it automatically levels off, so there is less shaping required. The shaping that is required can be done at a more leisurely pace, because the product has a longer drying time.

When the nails are dry, the surface has a tacky, gummy residue. As you refine the nails, this residue rolls off. The refining process is finished when the product stops rolling off.

You cannot mix traditional acrylics and odorless products because they are not chemically compatible.

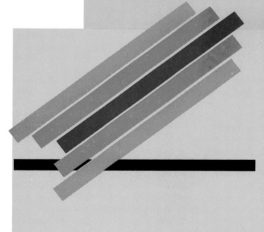

Practice Makes Perfect

Acrylic nail services do take a little longer than other nail services, but don't be tempted to cut corners for the sake of speed. Instead, work smarter by avoiding some errors common to beginning nail technicians. To avoid lifting, prime the nail according to the manufacturer's instructions. To create a professional-looking nail, pre-shape your form and use two for strength until you become accustomed to doing acrylic nails. To avoid creating an unnatural-looking bump in the center of the nail, wipe your brush frequently on a terrycloth towel so that no dried product remains on your brush. Do not use paper towel because small bits of paper can stick to your brush. To avoid overworking the product, practice making accurate movements. The more you practice, the more precise your work will be.

Review Questions

1. List the supplies needed for acrylic nail application.
2. Briefly describe the chemistry of acrylic nails.
3. Describe the procedure for the application of acrylic nails over forms.
4. Describe the safety precautions for applying primer.
5. Describe the procedure for applying acrylic nails over tips.
6. How does the procedure for acrylic nail application over bitten nails differ from other acrylic nail procedures?
7. Describe the two basic types of maintenance for acrylic nails.
8. Describe the proper procedure for acrylic removal.
9. Explain how the application of odorless acrylics differs from the application of traditional acrylics.

CHAPTER 14

The Creative Touch

LEARNING OBJECTIVES

After you have studied this chapter, you should be able to:
1. Describe the two basic types of gels.
2. List the supplies needed for light-gel application.
3. Demonstrate the proper procedure and precautions for light-cured gel application.
4. Demonstrate the proper procedure and precautions for light-gel cured application over forms.
5. Demonstrate the proper procedure and precautions for no-light gel application.
6. Demonstrate one nail art application.

Introduction

This chapter is an introduction to the creative nail services you can perform for clients. By now you have mastered the basic skills you need to become a professional nail technician; however, you have just begun to explore the world of nail art and new innovative services. During your career you should always seek out information about new products through manufacturer's seminars, continuing education, and professional associations. The more you learn, the better you will be able to please and excite your clients.

The following pages introduce the services you can perform with gels and nail art. *Gels* are strong, durable artificial nails that are brushed on the nail plate like polish. They have a chemical consistency very similar to the consistency of acrylic nails, but they require a separate catalyst to harden. There are two types of gels. *Light-cured gels* harden when they are exposed to a special light source—either an ultraviolet light or a halogen light. *No-light* gels harden when a gel activator is sprayed or brushed on, or when they are soaked in water.

Gels are available in colors that need no polish. These nails look as if they have already been polished and stay the same color until the gel itself is removed. Polish may be worn over colored gels. When polish is removed, the gel color will remain the same. Colored gels are a great base for nail art.

Nail art offers endless opportunities for you to express your creativity and your client's unique personality. For example, you can create a nail extension with red gel, polish half of it with blue polish, and paint it with stars, stripes, cats eyes, or tiger lilies highlighted with a rhinestone dew drop. With a creative touch, your imagination and your client's desires are your only limits. (Fig. 14.1)

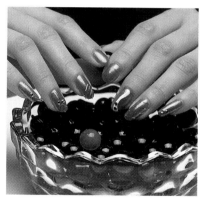

14.1 — Nail art

Light-Cured Gel on Tips or Natural Nails

SUPPLIES

In addition to the materials in your basic manicuring set-up, you will need the following items:

Light-cured gel.

Curing light. A box that has an *ultraviolet* or *halogen* bulb to cure or harden the gel nail. The type of light and the shape of the box varies from manufacturer to manufacturer.

Brush. Some nail technicians prefer to use a synthetic brush with small, flat, square bristles to hold and spread the gel.

Nail forms.
Primer (if recommended by gel manufacturer).
Block buffer.
Nail tips.
Adhesive.
Nail art supplies. (Fig. 14.2)

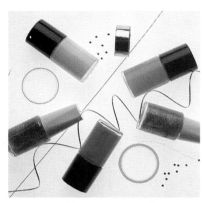

14.2 — Nail art materials: polish, foil, and striping tape

GEL APPLICATION PRE-SERVICE

1. Do your Pre-Service Sanitation procedure. (This procedure is described on pages 29–30.)
2. Set up your standard manicuring table. Place light-cured gel materials on your table.
3. Greet client and ask her to wash her hands with antibacterial soap. Dry hands thoroughly with a fresh towel.
4. Do client consultation, using health/record card to record responses and observations. Check for nail disorders and decide if it is safe and appropriate to perform a service on this client. If the client should not receive a service, explain your reasons and refer him or her to a doctor.

LIGHT-CURED GEL PROCEDURE

1. **Remove polish.** Begin with your client's left hand, little finger, and work toward the thumb. Then repeat on the right hand.
2. **Clean nails.** Ask client to dip nails in fingerbowl filled with antibacterial soap. Then use nail brush to clean nails over fingerbowl. Rinse nails briefly in clear water. Dry hands thoroughly with a fresh towel.
3. **Push back cuticles.** Use a cotton-tipped orangewood stick to gently push back cuticles.
4. **Buff nails to remove shine.** Buff lightly over nail plate with a medium/fine abrasive to remove the natural oil. Brush off filings.
5. **Apply nail antiseptic.** Apply nail antiseptic to nails. Begin with the little finger on the left hand and work toward the thumb.
6. **Apply tips if desired.** If your client wants tips, apply them according to the procedure described in Chapter 11.
7. **Apply primer if recommended by gel manufacturer.** If primer is recommended by the manufacturer of the gel you are using, put on plastic gloves and a pair of safety glasses. Offer a pair of safety glasses to your client. Apply a dot of the primer recommended by the manufacturer on nail plate with a cotton-tipped orangewood stick. Allow primer to dry to a chalky white.

PROCEDURAL TIP

▶ The procedure recommended for applying and curing gel varies from one manufacturer to another. Some systems recommend applying gel to four nails on one hand and curing, and then repeating this procedure on the other hand before applying and curing gel on the thumbnails. Other manufacturers provide light sources that cure only one finger at a time. Be sure to follow the instructions recommended by the manufacturer of the system you are using.

8. **Apply gel.** Brush gel onto entire nail. Cover with a thin, even layer as you would nail polish. Do not brush on cuticle because gel will lift. (Fig. 14.3)

9. **Cure gel.** Place nails under light source and set timer for time recommended by manufacturer. (Figs. 14.4, 14.5)

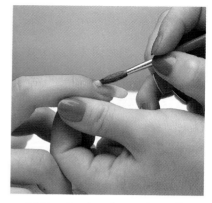

14.3 — Apply gel to entire nail.

PROCEDURAL TIP

▶ During the procedure keep brush and gel away from light to prevent hardening of gel.

10. **Repeat steps 8 and 9 on the other hand.**

11. **Apply second coat of gel to the first hand.** Apply gel in a thin and even coat that looks like a glossy top coat. Do not leave any imperfections in application because the finished nail will not be smooth.

12. **Cure gel.**

13. **Repeat steps 11 and 12 on the other hand.**

14. **Repeat steps 11–13.**

15. **Clean nails.** Wipe nails with alcohol or manufacturer's suggested cleanser to remove residue and tackiness on cured acrylic nails. Cured nails have a shiny gloss that needs no buffing if applied smoothly.

16. **Apply cuticle oil.** Rub cuticle oil into surrounding skin and nail surface.

17. **Apply hand lotion and massage hand and arm.**

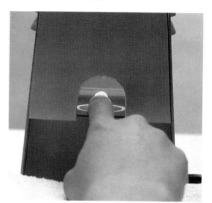

14.4 — Cure gel.

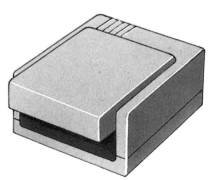

14.5 — Ultraviolet light source

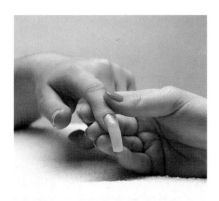

14.6 — Finished gel nail

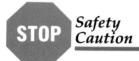

Inadequately shielded ultraviolet lamps can damage eyes and skin.

18. **Clean nails.** Ask client to dip nails in fingerbowl filled with antibacterial soap. Then use nail brush to clean nails over fingerbowl. Rinse with water and dry thoroughly.

19. **Apply polish.**

GEL APPLICATION POST-SERVICE

Your light-cured gel service is complete. Follow the post-service procedure described below. (Fig. 14.6)

1. **Make another appointment.** Schedule another appointment with your client to maintain the service she has just received or to perform another service.

2. **Suggest retail products.** Suggest that your client buy products necessary to maintain her nails throughout the week. Polish, lotion, top coat, etc. are valuable maintenance tools for her to have.

3. **Clean up around your table.** Take the time to restore the basic set-up of your table.

4. **Discard used materials.** Place all used materials in the plastic bag at the side of the table. Empty the bag frequently when you are doing gel nails.

5. **Sanitize table and implements.** Perform the complete pre-service sanitation procedure. In most states, this procedure calls for 20 minutes of proper sanitation before implements can be used on the next client.

Light-Cured Gel over Forms

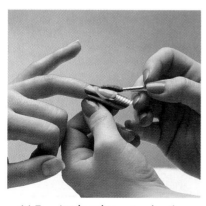

14.7 — Apply gel to natural nail.

Clients who want to strengthen and lengthen their natural nails with a light-weight artificial nail may choose gel nails over forms.

1. **Complete gel application pre-service.** Place light-cured gel supplies on your manicuring table.

2. **Apply nail forms.** Fit forms onto all ten fingers just as you would for acrylic nails over forms.

3. **Apply gel to natural nail.** Apply gel first to the natural nail only, not the nail form. (Fig. 14.7)

4. **Cure gel.** (Fig. 14.8)

5. **Create free edge.** Apply gel to the nail form to create a free edge. (Fig. 14.9)

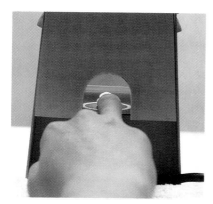
14.8 — Cure gel.

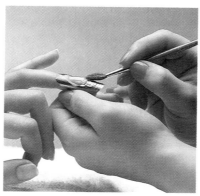
14.9 — Create free edge.

6. **Cure gel.**

7. **Apply gel to entire nail.** Apply gel to entire nail—both the natural nail and the free edge.

8. **Cure gel.**

9. **Remove forms.**

10. **Shape free edge.**

11. **Apply gel to entire nail without form.**

12. **Cure gel.**

13. **Remove residue.** Wipe nails with alcohol or manufacturer's suggested cleanser to remove residue and tackiness on cured acrylic nails. Cured nails have a shiny gloss that needs no buffing if applied smoothly.

14. **Apply cuticle oil.** Rub cuticle oil into surrounding skin and nail surface.

15. **Apply hand cream and massage hand and arm.**

16. **Clean nails.** Ask client to dip nails in fingerbowl filled with antibacterial soap. Then use nail brush to clean nails over fingerbowl. Rinse with water and dry thoroughly.

17. **Apply polish.**

18. **Complete gel application post-service.** (Fig. 14.10)

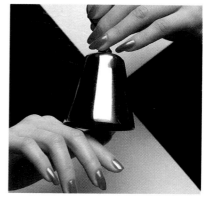
14.10 — Finished gel nails

No-Light Gel Application

No-light gels come in many varieties with different curing agents. Some are soaked in water and some are sprayed with an activator. The following is a generic procedure designed to show you how no-light gels are applied. For actual application you will need to follow your maufacturer's instructions carefully.

1. **Complete gel application pre-service.**
2. **Remove polish.** Begin with your client's left hand, little finger, and work toward the thumb. Then repeat on the right hand.
3. **Clean nails.** Ask client to dip nails in fingerbowl filled with antibacterial soap. Then use nail brush to clean nails over fingerbowl. Rinse nails briefly in clear water.
4. **Push back cuticles.** Use a cotton-tipped orangewood stick to gently push back cuticles.
5. **Buff nails to remove shine.** Buff lightly over nail plate with a medium/fine abrasive to remove the natural oil. Brush off filings.
6. **Apply nail antiseptic.** Apply nail antiseptic to nails. Begin with the little finger on the left hand and work toward the thumb.
7. **Apply tips if desired.** If your client wants tips, apply them according to the procedure described in Chapter 11.
8. **Apply gel.** Use brush to paint on gel or use bottle to spread a thin coat of gel onto entire nail. Apply gel to the five nails of one hand. Do not brush on cuticle because gel will lift.

PROCEDURAL TIP

▶ *Some gels run and must be applied and cured one finger at a time. Be guided by manufacturer's instructions.*

9. **Cure gel with activator or water.** *Activator-Cured:* Spray or brush gel activator (also called adhesive dryer) onto nail plate. If you use a spray, hold it at least 8 inches away from the client's nails to reduce the chance of having your client experience a heat reaction from the activator. *Water-Cured:* Immerse nails in lukewarm water for 2–5 minutes, depending on manufacturer's directions.
10. **Repeat steps 8 and 9 on the other hand.**
11. **Apply second coat of gel and cure if necessary.** With no-light gels, a second application of gel may not be necessary. Follow your manufacturer's directions for correct application.

12. **Shape and refine nails.** Shape and refine the entire surface of the nail with a medium/fine abrasive. Use a light touch to remove any imperfections.

13. **Buff nail.** Buff nail with block buffer to shine.

14. **Apply cuticle oil.** Rub cuticle oil into surrounding skin and nail surface.

15. **Apply hand cream and massage hand and arm.**

16. **Clean nails.** Ask client to dip nails in fingerbowl filled with antibacterial soap. Then use nail brush to clean nails over fingerbowl. Rinse with water and dry thoroughly.

17. **Apply polish.**

18. **Complete gel application post-service.**

Gel Maintenance and Removal

GEL MAINTENANCE

Both light-cured and non-light-cured gels should be maintained every two to three weeks, depending on how fast the client's nails grow. Use a medium abrasive file and buff entire nail to remove shine. Eliminate regrowth ledge by gliding file over ledge area. Hold file flat at ledge, not at an angle, because this can make a groove and damage the natural nail plate. Shape nail and blend it into the natural nail. Continue buffing until there is no line between hardened gel and natural nail plate. Be careful not to damage the natural nail plate by buffing too roughly. When the nail is smooth, follow the procedure for the application of gel on natural nails.

GEL REMOVAL

Soak client's nails for a few minutes in small glass bowl containing enough acetone (or gel remover recommended by gel manufacturer) to cover nails. Use orangewood stick to slide off softened tip. Gently buff natural nail with fine block buffer to remove the glue residue. Condition cuticle and surrounding skin with cuticle oil and lotion.

Creating Nail Art

Nail art is an exciting and creative part of a nail technician's job. It turns nails into small canvases on which you can paint pictures, create designs, and make collages with tiny gems, foils, tapes, or whatever your client will wear.

This section will provide you with a brief introduction to creating artistic nails with gems, foils, tape, and air brushing. You will also learn the procedures for creating holly berries, a design called "the sweep," and marbled gold.

If you are interested in providing nail art services for your clients, you might want to wear artistic designs on your own nails. This will give your clients a chance to see examples of the type of work you can do. (Fig. 14.11)

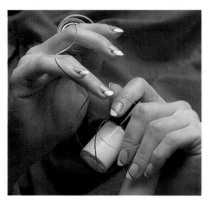

14.11 — Wear artistic designs on your own nails.

You may not have to schedule extra time to do nail art because often only one finger is done. Creating nail art on one finger takes only 2 or 3 minutes; but all ten fingers or a very complex design will take longer.

Every nail technician is an artist. This is your chance to be creative. The colors and designs in the world around you will give you ideas for new art. Even mistakes you make could be the beginning of a new creation. Make mistakes into some abstract design. Don't forget there is always nail polish remover to wipe the nail canvases clean so you can start again.

GEMS

Tiny rhinestones are popular nail art materials. They come in different shapes, colors, and sizes. **Gems** give sparkle to a design and add texture.

Use a wet orangewood stick to pick up small gems on the shiny side of the stone. Put them on while the top coat of the polish is still tacky so gems will adhere. Allow nail to dry and apply another top coat over gems. Reapply top coat every three or four days to seal gem to nail and revitalize the shine.

You can use either tweezers or an orangewood stick to pick up large gems. If you use the orangewood stick, dip it in top coat and touch the shiny surface of the gem with the sticky tip of the orangewood stick.

Use acetone to remove gems from your clients' nails. These gems can be reused if the silver backing stays in place. If the silver backing comes off a gem, it must be thrown away because it will no longer reflect color.

STRIPING TAPE

Striping tape comes in rolls of different colors, although silver, gold, and black are the most popular. Tape has a tacky backing and is

The Teen Scene

Cash in on the teen market for nail art and nail jewelry by throwing a teen party. Schedule it right before the prom, graduation, or a major holiday. Make your prices reasonable and check teen magazines and music videos to be sure you're offering art and jewelry that appeal to the teen market. Advertise the event locally, offer refreshments, and get a stylist to give a free mini hair styling lesson. Offer a free trial service or very inexpensive art on a single nail. Your teen clients can opt to purchase more art, a different design, or nail jewelry. What's your key to success? The teens themselves. Involve them in the planning. If you don't know any teens, ask your local high school to recommend an "advisory board" and offer members free nail services for their help.

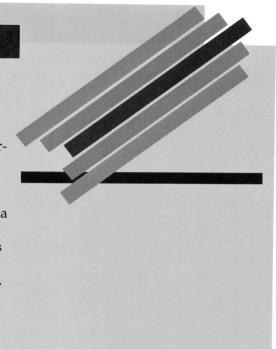

stuck to a dry, polished nail. Lift the edge of the tape when it is on the nail and, using nippers, cut it 1/16 inch away from cuticle and free edge. This will prevent the tape from peeling and rolling off the nail. Seal tape on nail with top coat and reapply top coat every three to four days.

FOIL

Foil is very fragile leafing that is available in gold, silver, and copper. It comes in sheets that are packaged approximately ten to a bag. Sheets should be stored in the bag to protect them from cracking. Use tweezers to remove the piece you need. Put the leaf on your table, and rip off little pieces with tweezers or an orangewood stick. Put these small pieces of foil on the tacky top coat.

Foil leaf is used to accentuate parts of a nail. As an example, if you paint half a nail red and the other half black, you can use gold foil to highlight the black portion of each nail or the line between the two colors. Seal the foil with a top coat and reapply the top coat every three to four days.

PROCEDURE FOR HOLLY BERRIES

The procedure for holly berries is easy to learn if you follow each step carefully. Your clients will enjoy wearing holly berry nail art when they participate in holiday gatherings.

1. Polish entire nail bright red.
2. Use a 000 art brush and paint a small, green flattened diamond shape. (Fig. 14.12)
3. Connect two more small diamond shapes to the first. (Fig. 14.13)
4. Design two additional holly leaves in a semicircle. (Fig. 14.14)

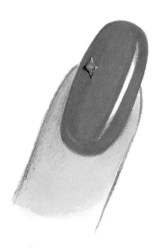 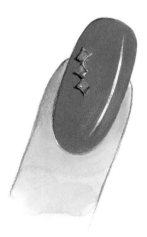 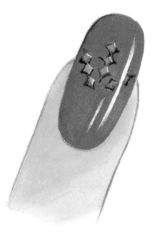

14.12 — Paint small flat diamond.

14.13 — Add two or more diamonds.

14.14 — Design holly leaves.

5. Place three beads of gold metallic polish and three red rhinestones at the center of the leaves to create shiny holly berries. (Fig. 14.15)

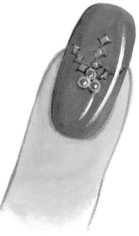

14.15 — Apply gold beads to make holly berries.

6. Dot leaves and berries with gold polish for highlights. (Fig. 14.16)
7. Brush leaves and berries with a top coat for shine and protection. Repeat top coat every three days.

PROCEDURE FOR "THE SWEEP"

The procedure for the sweep will show you how to make a two-color nail art design that will be the perfect complement to your clients' "spectator pump" shoes. It is also a design that can be worn well with any two-tone fashion look.

1. Polish entire nail one color.
2. Brush on white polish diagonally from left to right. Beginning at the center of nail along left sidewall, apply it on an angle across the free edge. (Fig. 14.17)
3. Use black polish to paint a narrow strip of black along the free edge, on top of the white polish. Start at the center sidewall and paint to the center of the free edge.
4. Use orangewood stick and sweep black polish onto white polish in light feather strokes. (Fig. 14.18)
5. Let dry, then brush entire nail with top coat.

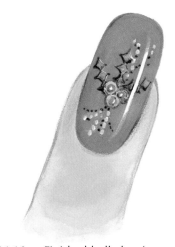

14.16 — Finished holly berries

PROCEDURE FOR MARBLED GOLD

Marbled gold nail art adds sparkle and flair to your clients' nails. With this procedure you can select complementary nail polish colors that coordinate perfectly with your clients' fashion choices. When these colors are swirled together, they add a very interesting touch to any fashion look.

1. Polish entire nail in a color, for example, pink.
2. Puddle complementary colors, such as white, gold, and deep pink, on the top half of nail at an angle. (Fig. 14.19)
3. Use orangewood stick and lightly swirl colors together on half of the nail. (Fig. 14.20)

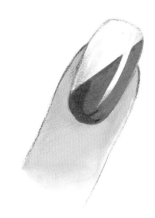

14.17 — Brush on white polish diagonally.

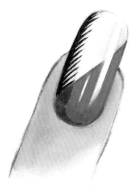

14.18 — Finished sweep

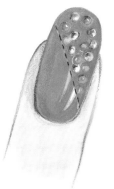

14.19 — Puddle complementary colors on top half of nail.

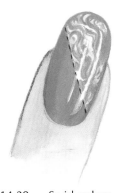

14.20 — Swirl colors.

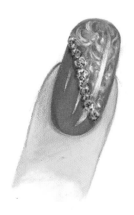

14.21 — Finished marbled gold

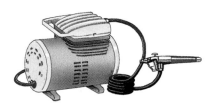

14.22 — Air brush machine

4. Let nail dry and apply top coat.
5. Pick up small pieces of gold foil and place them along the line between the marbled top half of the nail and the solid color at the bottom half of the nail. (Fig. 14.21)
6. Apply top coat for protection and shine.

USING AN AIR BRUSH

An *air brush* is a compressor that pushes air through a brush. When paint is pushed through the brush, shades and textures of color are created. The dual-action air brush is the most common type used for nail art. The basic operation of the dual-action air brush is simple. Air is released when you press down on the lever. Paint is released when you pull back on the lever. The lever controls the force and width of the paint spray. You can release a very fine dusting of paint, a heavy spray, and everything in between. (Fig. 14.22)

You can learn to control air and paint by practicing with the lever. With good control, you will be able to create the effects you want without spraying your hands or your client's hands. As a general rule, use less paint for better results.

You can use stencils to create unique designs or simply use your imagination. If you use acrylic water-based paints, the designs must have a top coat to preserve them or they will wash off with water.

An air brush must be cleaned when you move from one color to the next, especially if the second color is lighter. It is cleaned with air brush cleaner. Always release your last spray of paint onto a mat when you are emptying it for cleaning.

You will have to clean the air brush fewer times if you start a design with the lightest color and systematically add darker colors.

Review Questions

1. Describe the two basic types of gels.
2. List the supplies needed for light-gel application.
3. Describe the proper procedure and precautions for light-cured gel application.
4. Describe the proper procedure and precautions for light-gel application over forms.
5. Describe no-light gel application.
6. Why should you develop nail art skills?

PART V

THE BUSINESS OF NAIL TECHNOLOGY

- *Chapter 15 - Salon Business*
- *Chapter 16 - Selling Nail Products and Services*

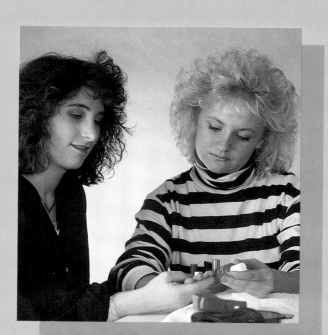

CHAPTER 15

Salon Business

LEARNING OBJECTIVES

After you have studied this chapter, you should be able to:
1. Discuss the advantages and disadvantages of working in a full-service salon.
2. Discuss the advantages and disadvantages of working in a nails-only salon.
3. List ten questions you will need to ask before deciding what salon is right for you.
4. List eight questions that will help you determine if a salon has safe working conditions.
5. Explain the difference between income and expenses and give two examples of each.
6. List the practical uses for business records that are required by local, state, and federal laws.
7. List the types of information that a salon can gather by keeping accurate business records.
8. Discuss the advantages of keeping proper service, inventory, and personal appointment records.
9. List the guidelines that should be followed in booking appointments.

Introduction

You are training to become part of a $2 billion nail care industry. If you want to be financially successful in this business, you must know more than how to give clients manicures, pedicures, or artificial nail services. You should also be a good business person. From the moment you receive a job offer, you have to negotiate how much money you are paid. When you develop a clientele, you will handle tips and, possibly, a commission.

If you someday decide to open your own salon, you will be responsible for the complicated business of renting or buying a shop, and paying expenses such as electricity, telephone, advertising, safety systems, employee salaries, and taxes. You may be an expert nail technician, but if you can't handle the business part of nail care, you will not make as much money as nail technicians who can.

Your Working Environment

Good business sense begins with the decisions you make when you look for your first job. Should you work for a full-service or a nails-only salon? There are advantages and disadvantages to each choice.

THE FULL-SERVICE SALON

Unless they are large and very successful, *full-service salons* often employ only one nail technician. The arrangement is a convenient one for both the nail technician and the salon. You automatically get all of the nail-care business in the salon, and your services make it convenient for clients to have their nails done when they are there for hair-care or skin-care services. You might make arrangements with the salon to attract clients by offering them special rates for nail care when they have other services performed.

On the other hand, at a full-service salon, there won't be other nail technicians with whom to share ideas and experience. There also won't be someone to fill in for you when you are sick or on vacation. If the salon is a traditional one, you may be limited in the variety of artificial nail services that you are allowed to perform. (Fig. 15.1)

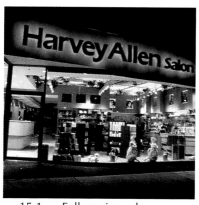

15.1 — Full-service salon

THE NAILS-ONLY SALON

In a *nails-only salon* you will work with several other nail technicians. In addition to having the opportunity to share ideas and experiences, you could increase your business by serving their clients when they are sick, on vacation, or retire. (Fig. 15.2)

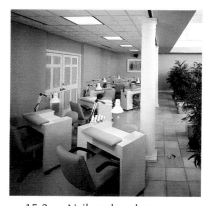

15.2 — Nails-only salon

The client who patronizes a nails-only salon may take nail care more seriously than clients who have their nails done in full-service salons. Your clients may have special nail problems, or want more creative artificial nail services. If this is the case, you will gain valuable experience. A nails-only salon is a good place for a nail technician to establish a serious clientele. On the other hand, there could be competition for clients in a nails-only salon where there are many nail technicians.

MAKING YOUR DECISION

Before you make a decision about what salon is right for you, visit several full-service and several nails-only salons. Observe the working environment and decide which feels comfortable to you.

You will want to consider the following factors in deciding on the salon that is right for you:

1. Will the salon provide additional training for you or encourage you to attend training outside the salon?
2. Will the salon help you build a clientele? Will they spend money on advertising low-price specials? Will they refer customers to you?
3. Will you be considered an employee, or will you be an independent contractor who rents a booth? If you are an independent contractor, what are the terms of the booth rental?
4. If you are an employee, how will the salon pay you? Will you receive a weekly salary or salary plus commission? Will you receive a commission on retail products sold? Is there a regular salary review?
5. Will the salon provide nail-care products or will you have to bring your own?
6. Does the salon offer benefits such as medical, liability, life insurance, or paid sick days?
7. Are there fixed or flexible working hours?
8. What is the dress code?
9. Does the salon close for a regular vacation period, or does each employee take a separate vacation?
10. What is the salon's reputation? There is an advantage to working in a successful "upscale" salon where you can make good contacts and learn valuable tricks of the trade from your employer and coworkers.
11. Does the salon have safe working conditions?
    a) Does it have proper ventilation, like an exhaust system to the outside?
    b) Does it provide separate refrigerators for food and nail product storage?

c) Are MSDS sheets on display or within easy access to employees?

d) Are work stations well-equipped and clean, with plastic disposal bags that can be closed?

e) Are nail technicians required to wear dust masks?

f) Are nail technicians required to wear safety glasses?

g) Are aerosol cans used or are safer application methods used, such as pumps or drop-on products?

h) Are salon workers ready for emergencies? Are the telephone numbers for poison control, the hospital, paramedics, the fire station, or the police posted in a visible place?

Keeping Good Personal Records

Although you may not be required to keep business records for your salon, you will want to develop a simple and efficient system for keeping track of your own income and expenses. You will also want to save all of your check stubs, cancelled checks, receipts, and invoices. Basically, *income* is the money you make and *expenses* are what you spend. Another valuable personal record is your appointment calendar.

INCOME

To keep a correct, conscise, and complete record of your income, you should create a form with room to list each source of income. It might include salary, commission from services, commission from retail products sold, and tips.

EXPENSES

Your expenses working in the salon could include equipment, supplies, magazines or books that explain techniques, comfortable shoes, uniforms (if required), and tuition for special courses on nail techniques.

APPOINTMENTS

Use a personal appointment calendar to help you arrange your work time. If you keep this calendar with you, you can plan each day's schedule before you arrive at the salon. You will know who your clients are, when each one will arrive, and the services you will perform. With this information, you can prepare all your supplies ahead of time, so you are more efficient.

Understanding Salon Business Records

Most salons use the services of an accountant to help them keep accurate records that meet the requirements of local, state, and federal laws. These records are used to:

1. Determine income, expenses, and profit or loss.
2. Prove the value of your clientele or the worth of the salon to prospective buyers.
3. Get a bank loan.
4. Compute income tax, social security, unemployment, and disability insurance, among others.

Businesses hold daily sales slips, the appointment book, and the petty cash book for at least one year. The payroll book, canceled checks, monthly and yearly records, and service and inventory records are usually held for at least seven years for tax purposes. (Fig. 15.3)

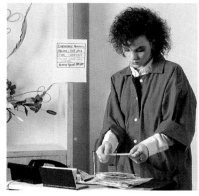

15.3 — Keep accurate and neat business records.

USING BUSINESS RECORDS

Accurate records will help you and your employer gather the following valuable information:

1. **Profit and loss comparisons with other weeks, months, or years.** As an example, over a period of time, you can see which are the slow months and which are the busiest in your business. This will allow you to cut expenses by not being overstocked during slow months, and being fully stocked during busy periods. You can also schedule vacations or renovations during the slow months and have a full staff and full service during the busy months.
2. **Changes in demands for services.** If the demand for a service is growing, your salon may choose to hire more nail technicians to service this growing demand.
3. **Inventory.** If you keep accurate records of inventory, you can cut costs by keeping the appropriate stock levels. This means that you are neither overstocked nor running short of supplies needed for services. Daily inventory records also help you quickly detect any loss of stock from theft.
4. **Net income.** Net income refers to all the income you make less all the expenses. Accurate net income records can help you establish the net worth of the business at the end of the year.
5. **Materials and supply levels.** Records will help you compare the use of materials and supplies with the services rendered to make sure that neither too much nor too little is being used.

KEEPING CLIENT RECORDS

A *client service record* lists services rendered and merchandise sold to each client. All service records should contain the name and address of the client, date, amount charged, product used, results obtained, and client's preferences and tastes. Most salons use a card file system or a memorandum book to keep service records. With the service record for each client should be any release statements that he or she has signed. Service records are especially valuable if another nail technician has to fill in for a client's usual nail technician. If the client's usual service is explained in detail on the card, it can be done accurately and efficiently.

The client health/record card lists clients' personal information, such as what types of jobs they have, what hobbies they have and what sports they enjoy. It is a good idea to start your day by reading the records of clients scheduled for services during the day. Your clients will be happy to know you remembered the things that are important to them. See Chapter 8 for a complete discussion of client records.

KEEPING INVENTORY RECORDS

Keep a running inventory of all supplies. Classify them by use and retail value. Those used in the business are *consumption supplies*. Those that are sold to the customer are *retail supplies*.

Booking Appointments

The system used in your salon will determine whether you book appointments with clients or they are booked by a receptionist. Keeping a proper record of appointments will cut down on the confusion, annoyance, and stress of overbooking and help prevent clients from arriving at the wrong time and having to wait.

Regardless of who books the appointments, the following guidelines should be followed: (Fig. 15.4)

1. Always have a supply of appointment books, pencils, erasers, pens, a calendar, and a message pad.

2. Be prompt. Whether you are answering the phone or acknowledging your client's presence at the counter, try not to keep them waiting.

3. Identify both yourself and the salon by name when you answer the telephone.

4. Be pleasant. Let clients know you are pleased to talk with them.

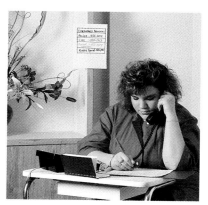

15.4 — Keep an accurate record of appointments.

5. Make sure to take the following information when a client calls to make an appointment: client's name and phone number, type of service to be performed, date, and time of appointment. Repeat the information to the client to be sure you are correct, then block out the amount of time needed to perform the service.
6. Speak clearly. Don't mumble or shout. Use correct English and avoid slang.
7. Be tactful and courteous when speaking. Refer to clients by their last name.
8. If you are busy enough to have appointments made in advance, it is a good practice to call your clients the night before the appointment to remind them and confirm the time. This will reduce your number of no-shows.
9. Always ask your clients at the end of their appointment if they wish to reschedule.

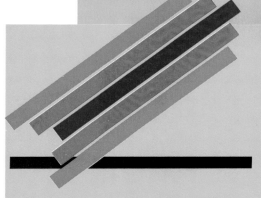

Added Value

In a competitive world, it's the little extras that make you stand out. Here are a few suggestions to add extra value to your nail service:

- Complimentary jewelry cleaning. Sparkling clean jewelry looks great with a fresh manicure. To offer free jewelry cleaning, simply let your client's jewelry soak in jewelry cleaner while you work on their nails.
- Conversation pits. Arrange manicuring tables so that clients can visit while you work. Encourage friends to book appointments together.
- Aromatherapy hand massage. You can offer a free three-minute hand massage with a manicure or offer one free during downtime to promote added services. Exfoliate your clients' hands, then massage in aromatherapy oils.
- Winter moisturizer and hot-mit treatments. While clients are waiting, offer free moisturizer and hot-mit treatments to warm their hands and speed waiting time.

Advertising Yourself

The first thing you might want to do when you begin a job in the salon is to make a list of every service you offer. Write a brief description of the service, length of time needed to perform it, and the cost of the service.

A copy of your service list should be kept near the appointment book so there will be no confusion among your clients about these facts. Give your coworkers a copy of your list of services and encourage them to offer your services to their clients.

Collecting Payment for Services

In some salons, the nail technician collects payments from clients. In others, the receptionist handles all payments. In either case, you will probably be required to prepare a ticket detailing the services you have performed for that client. The ticket should include the client's name, the date, the service provided, and the cost. The ticket will make it clear to clients what they are paying for and provide an accurate record of the transaction.

Do not offer reduced prices to special clients. This can lead to a difficult situation if your other clients are denied a price reduction.

Review Questions

1. What are the advantages and disadvantages of working in a full-service salon?
2. What are the advantages and disadvantages of working in a nails-only salon?
3. What are ten questions that will help you determine if a salon is right for you?
4. What are eight questions that will help you determine if a salon has safe working conditions?
5. Explain the difference between income and expenses and give two examples of each.
6. List four practical uses for business records that are required by local, state, and federal laws.
7. List five types of information that a salon can gather by keeping accurate business records.
8. Discuss the advantages of keeping proper service, inventory, and personal appointment records.
9. List nine guidelines that should be followed in booking appointments.

CHAPTER 16

Selling Nail Products and Services

LEARNING OBJECTIVES

After you have studied this chapter, you should be able to:
1. List the basic steps in selling.
2. Describe the difference between product features and benefits.
3. Demonstrate your ability to turn product features into benefits.
4. List the questions you should try to answer as you determine your client's needs and wants.
5. Explain how you can sell while you work.
6. List and describe the steps in closing the sale.

Introduction

If you want to be a successful nail technician, you need to be a good salesperson too. You are responsible for selling both nail services and the products that will help your clients maintain those services. You will be successful if you reach one basic selling goal—to meet the needs of your clients.

The five basic steps in meeting your clients' needs and selling your products and services are described in this chapter. The basic steps to selling include:

1. Know your products and services.
2. Know what your client needs and wants.
3. Present your products and services.
4. Answer your client's questions and objections properly.
5. Close the sale.

Know Your Products and Services

In the nail salon, products and services are very closely related. When you perform a nail service for your client, you select the products that are best for that person. Then you use them to perform a service that meets your client's needs and wants.

When you have finished with the nail service, you sell your client the products needed to maintain the service between visits to the salon.

There are two ways to know your products and services. One way is to know the features, and the other way is to know the benefits.

FEATURES

A *feature* is a specific fact about a product or service that describes it. Read labels, product bulletins, and industry literature to learn the features of your nail products. You look for information such as the ingredients your products contain, safety precautions you should follow when using them, how to apply them, and how to maintain them. Features of nail services include the procedures and how long they take to perform, the chemicals used, how much the services cost, what effect they have on the clients' nails, and how often they need maintenance.

The features of colored gel nails over tips include the fact that they are durable, lightweight, and come in a variety of colors. Light-cured gels take about 30 minutes to perform, use acrylic-based gel with a special light source, will not harm healthy nails, and need maintenance every two to three weeks. (Fig. 16.1)

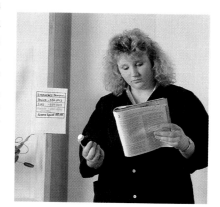

16.1 — Read about your retail products.

BENEFITS

The *benefits* of a product or service are what it will do for your client or how it will fulfill your client's needs and wants. The benefits of colored gel nails over tips are long, beautiful nails that save you both time and money. They give you nails that always look freshly polished, are lightweight and comfortable to wear, and require maintenance every two or three weeks instead of once a week.

You will be a good salesperson when you can turn the features of your products and services into benefits that meet the needs and desires of your clients.

Know What Your Client Needs and Wants

It is important to know your clients' nail needs if you want to sell them nail products and services that meet those needs. You can discover those needs during the client consultation (see Chapter 8).

As you observe your client and communicate with him or her, you will want to answer questions such as these:

1. **Does your client have special nail problems?** Clients with nail problems will need special nail services. Does your client have short bitten nails or nails that crack and tear easily? These clients may need services that strengthen or cover up their natural nails.

2. **What is your client's lifestyle?** The kind of life your client leads will determine what type of nail services they need. A business person may want nails that have a well-groomed look and are short and polished in a pale conservative color. A jewelry or cosmetics salesperson may want long, acrylic nails. A gardener or pianist might need short, natural-looking nails. A quilter might need short nails but want them polished in the latest fashion color. Be sure you give your clients the services and products that suit their activities and image. (Fig. 16.2)

   Nail "look" is one important consideration, but there are others. Wearability is another. A client whose hands are in water frequently may ask you for linen wraps. You would caution that client against linen wraps because they retain water and the dampness encourages the growth of mold and fungus on the wrap. You might suggest another service that would be more appropriate for this client, such as acrylic or gel nails.

3. **Is your client preparing for a special occasion?** A client who is going to a wedding might want nails that are the same color as the dress she is wearing. A client who is going on a job

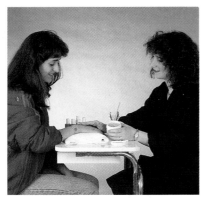

16.2 — Determine which services or products best suit your clients by discussing their lifestyles with them.

interview will probably want nails that look natural but well groomed. If your client is wearing a witch's costume to a Halloween party, she might want extra long acrylic nails painted black.

Present Your Products and Services

There are two powerful opportunities to sell your products and services to your clients. One way is while you are performing the service. The other way is to have the products and services displayed attractively near your work station.

SELL WHILE YOU WORK

When you are performing a service, tell your clients what you are doing, what products you are using, and why. If one of the procedures, such as nail filing and polish touch-up, can be done by your clients, suggest the type of abrasive and polish they should buy and tell them how to use the products.

While you are giving one service to a client, discuss other services and the features, benefits, and costs of each. If you are giving an acrylic nail service, compare it with linen wraps or gel nails. Your clients may want to try other services in the future.

DISPLAY A LIST OF YOUR SERVICES

Have your service list prominently displayed near your table. The card should be attractive and clear. It should list your services and the cost of each. You may put in other information you think would be helpful to your clients, such as length of time for each service, its features, and its benefits.

DISPLAY YOUR PRODUCTS

Display the nail products sold by your salon attractively and in view of your clients when they are having a service performed. Have written promotional materials about the products within easy reach of your clients so they can take information with them. Also, have free samples of nail products, when possible, and encourage your clients to take some and try them.

Don't pass up the opportunity to sell your clients polish, top coat, hand cream, polish remover, cuticle oil, and other products they will need to maintain their nail services between visits to the salon.

Home Care Kits Bring You Profits

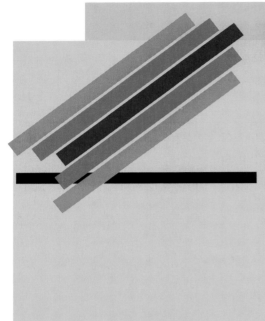

Selling a bottle of nail polish brings you additional income; selling products in "pre-packaged" groupings brings you super profits. Create home care kits around the services you provide. The home care kit for clients who get nail tips should include emergency nail glue, touch-up polish, a nail file, buffer, and non-acetone remover. For routine hand care, substitute a hand lotion for the nail glue. A home care kit for pedicures should include a foot file or pumice stone, an antifungal spray, sloughing lotion, conditioning lotion, and foot bath lotion, or salts for soaking tired feet. With a little imagination, you can also create kits for special occasions. Bridal touch-up kits, holiday stocking stuffers, and travel nail kits will give your clients the nail care products they need and bring you profits at the same time.

Answer Questions and Objections

Be ready to answer any questions or objections your clients have about your products and services. (Fig. 16.3)

QUESTIONS

Clients may want to know what type of polish has the most unusual colors, how nail art is done and what materials are used, or how long a service takes. They may want to know the advantages and disadvantages of a service or what they should do when their nail breaks. Be as knowledgeable as you can about your products and services, but don't be afraid to say you don't know the answer and will find it for your client.

OBJECTIONS

Don't be afraid of client objections to a product or service. A client may object to the price, length of time a service takes, the results of a service, or the frequent maintenance of a particular service. Answer the objection honestly and pleasantly, describing the advantages of the product or service and weighing them against the disadvantages. When a client has valid objections to a product or service, suggest another option that will serve his or her needs better.

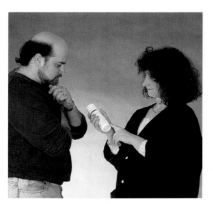

16.3 — Be ready to answer a client's questions about your products.

Close the Sale

When a client decides to buy a product or service, you have closed the sale. There are three basic steps to closing a sale for nail products and services: suggestion selling, wrap-up, and scheduling another appointment. (Fig. 16.4)

SUGGESTION SELLING

Suggestion selling occurs when you suggest products or services for your client to buy. You will be successful at suggestion selling when you can match your products and services with your client's needs and wants. After performing a service, you should try to sell your clients the products needed to maintain their nails until their next appointment.

You might suggest that a client buy an additional service before leaving. As an example, for clients with rough hands, suggest they get a paraffin waxing treatment to soften them.

16.4 — When a client decides to buy a product or service, you have closed the sale.

WRAP-UP

After the client has decided what to buy, you can close the sale by saying, "Should I wrap this up for you?" or "Will this be cash or charge?"

SCHEDULING ANOTHER APPOINTMENT

Before a client leaves the salon, schedule another appointment for maintenance of the service you just performed or for another service. Confirm future appointments by giving each client your business card with the date and time of the next appointment. Advance scheduling is a good way to build a steady, happy clientele.

Review Questions

1. What are the five basic steps in selling.
2. Describe the difference between product features and benefits.
3. Choose one of the nail services you have learned about in this book. Describe two features and two benefits of that service.
4. What are three questions you should try to answer as you determine your client's needs and wants?
5. Explain how you can sell while you work.
6. List and describe the three steps in closing the sale.

Answers to Review Questions

CHAPTER 1

1. What is salon conduct?

   Salon conduct is the way you act when working with clients, your employer, and coworkers in a salon.

2. Give ten examples of professional salon conduct toward clients.

   Examples of professional salon conduct toward clients are: 1) being on time; 2) being prepared; 3) planning your day; 4) arranging appointments carefully; 5) keeping clients informed of schedule changes; 6) being courteous; 7) performing all tasks willingly and efficiently; 8) communicating with clients; 9) never complaining or arguing with a client; 10) using good judgment; 11) never chewing gum, smoking, or eating where you can be seen by clients. (Only 10 are needed.)

3. Explain why a salon might lose clients if nail technicians do not exhibit professional salon conduct.

   A salon might lose clients if nail technicians do not exhibit professional salon conduct because clients want to be treated well. If you are late, or you seem disorganized or uncaring, clients might feel uncomfortable. Clients shouldn't feel that their appointments inconvenience you. Chewing gum, smoking, or eating in front of clients can annoy them. Smoking can also be potentially dangerous around chemicals.

4. Give ten examples of professional salon conduct toward employers and coworkers.

   Examples of professional salon conduct toward employers and coworkers are: 1) being willing to learn; 2) communicating; 3) giving credit to others; 4) respecting the opinions of coworkers; 5) taking the initiative; 6) using good judgment; 7) leaving personal problems at home; 8) never borrowing money from employers or coworkers; 9) promoting the salon; 10) developing your ability to sell.

5. Define professional ethics.

   Professional ethics is your sense of right and wrong when you interact with your clients, employer, and coworkers. The essential values in professional ethics are honesty, fairness, courtesy, and respect for the feelings and rights of others.

6. Give seven examples of professional ethics toward clients.

   Examples of professional ethics toward clients are: 1) suggesting services that meet clients' needs; 2) keeping your word and fulfilling all obligations; 3) treating all clients fairly; 4) following state regulations for sanitation and safety; 5) being loyal; 6) not criticizing others; 7) not abandoning clients.

7. Give five examples of professional ethics toward employers and coworkers.

   Five examples of professional ethics toward employers and coworkers are: 1) being honest; 2) fulfilling obligations; 3) respecting the talents of your employer and coworkers; 4) not inviting criticism of coworkers; 5) never gossiping or starting rumors among coworkers.

8. Describe the type of appearance you should have as a professional nail technician.

   As a nail technician one should be clean and fresh, have fresh breath and healthy teeth, wear clean clothes that are appropriate for the salon, and pay attention to hair, skin, and nails.

9. Explain why a salon might lose clients if it employs nail technicians who have an unprofessional appearance.

   A salon might lose clients if it employs nail technicians who have an unprofessional appearance because, as a member of the beauty industry, a nail technician should be pleasant to be around. If you are not clean and pleasant smelling, clients may object to having you touch them while performing nail services.

CHAPTER 2

1. What are bacteria? What do bacteria look like?

   Bacteria are one-celled vegetable microorganisms that can only be seen through a microscope.

2. Are all bacteria harmful? Give examples to explain your answer.

   Not all bacteria are harmful. Nonpathogenic bacteria decompose matter. Some nonpathogenic bacteria help produce food and oxygen. Others are used to improve the fertility of soil.

3. What are the three main groups of pathogenic bacteria? Describe each of them.

   Three main groups of pathogenic bacteria are cocci, bacilli, and spirilla. Cocci are round, pus-producing bacteria. Bacilli are rod-shaped bacteria that produce diseases such as tetanus, influenza, typhoid, tuberculosis, and diphtheria. Spirilla are spiral or corkscrew-shaped bacteria.

4. Name and describe three types of cocci.

   Three types of cocci are: 1) staphylococci, which grow in clusters and are present in local infections such as absecesses, pustules, and boils. 2) streptococci, which grow in chains, cause strep throat and diseases that spread throughout the body such as blood poisoning and rheumatoid fever. 3) diplococci, which grow in pairs and cause pneumonia.

5. Describe the process of mitosis. Explain why it is important to bacteria growth.

   Mitosis is the crosswise division into halves of a mature cell. It forms two identical cells. Mitosis is important to bacteria growth because through mitosis, one bacterium can produce as many as 16 million bacteria in 12 hours.

6. Give examples of common infections caused by viruses.

   Examples of common infections caused by viruses include hepatitis, chicken pox, influenza, measles, mumps, and the common cold. These infections can be transferred through casual contact with an infected person.

7. Explain how it is possible to transfer AIDS in the salon.

   It is possible to transfer AIDS in the salon if you accidentally cut a client who is infected with AIDS, then transfer that blood to another client.

8. Describe the appearance of nail mold at its various stages of development.

   Nail mold in the early stages is seen as a yellow/green spot that becomes darker in advanced stages. Over a period of time its discoloration eventually becomes black. The nail will then soften and smell bad. Eventually the nail may fall off.

9. What is immunity? Name three types of immunity.

   Immunity is the ability of the body to resist disease and destroy microorganisms when they have entered the body. Three types of immunity are: 1) natural immunity; 2) naturally acquired immunity; 3) artificially acquired immunity.

10. Name five common sources of infection in the salon.

    Five common sources of infection in the salon are: 1) contaminated manicuring tools and equipment; 2) a client's nails, hands, and feet; 3) clients', coworkers', and your own mouth, nose, and eyes; 5) objects throughout the entire salon.

11. Explain four ways that you can fight infections within the salon.

    Four ways to fight infections within the salon are: 1) learning proper sanitation procedures and following them; 2) not working in contagious conditions; 3) not working near open wounds; 4) not causing wounds.

CHAPTER 3

1. What is the difference between sterilization and sanitation?

    Sterilization means to make something germ free by destroying all bacteria, whereas sanitation means to make clean and prevent germs from growing. Sanitary does not mean germ free.

2. Describe two methods of sanitation.

    Two methods for sanitation are: 1) by using physical agents such as ultraviolet rays, moist heat, and dry heat; 2) by using chemical agents such as alcohol, quats, and formalin.

3. List three types of equipment used to sanitize.

    Three types of equipment used to sanitize are: 1) wet sanitizer; 2) dry cabinet sanitizer; 3) ultraviolet ray electrical scrutinizer.

4. What are four different ways to sanitize with physical agents.

    Four different ways to sanitize with physical agents are: 1)ultraviolet rays; 2) moist heat; 3) boiling; 4) steaming.

5. Why isn't sterilization practical in a salon?

    Sterilization is not practical in a salon because it is only possible to have a sterile area if it is sealed off from everything including air and human contact. In a salon, the work area is in constant use and is exposed to air and humans.

6. What are three safety precautions to follow when using chemical agents for sanitation?

    Three safety precautions to follow when using chemical agents for sanitation are: 1) purchase chemicals in small quantities and store them in a cool, dry place; 2) weigh and measure chemicals carefully; 3) keep all containers labeled and under lock and key; 4) do not smell chemicals or solutions; 5) avoid spills when dissolving or diluting chemicals; 6) keep a complete first-aid kit on hand; 7) follow manufacturer's directions; 8) be sure to watch small children at your work station.

CHAPTER 4

1. Name five chemicals commonly used by nail technicians in the salon.

    Five chemicals commonly used by nail technicians in the salon are: 1) solvents; 2) liquid and powder for acrylic nails; 3) primer; 4) gel nail supplies; 5) adhesive dryer or gel activator; 6) glue. (Only five are needed.)

2. What are five early warning signs of overexposure to nail chemicals?

    Five early warning signs of overexposure include: 1) lightheadedness; 2) insomnia; 3) runny nose; 4) sore, dry nose; 5) watery eyes; 6) tingling toes; 7) tiredness all day; 8) irritability; 9) sluggishness; 10) breathing problems. (Only five are needed.)

3. What is an MSDS?

    An MSDS is a Material Safety Data Sheet. The MSDS informs salon employees of the potential hazards, proper handling, and signs of overexposure for any product.

4. What is meant by the term flashpoint?

    Flashpoint is the temperature at which a liquid will give off enough flammable vapor to ignite.

5. What are three ways that products can enter the body and cause harm.

    Three ways that products can enter the body and cause harm are through inhalation, skin contact, and ingestion.

6. What are five ways you can protect yourself and your clients when using chemicals?

    Five ways to protect yourself and clients when using chemicals are: 1) ventilate; 2) avoid sprayng products into the air; 3) keep products off skin; 4) wear a dust mask while filing; 5) wear safety glasses; 6) never wear contact lenses in the salon; 7) don't smoke in the salon; 8) never eat or drink in the salon area; 9) store and eat lunch in a separate area of the salon; 10) always wash your hands before eating; 11) label all containers; 12) store products in a cool area; 13) throw out trash regularly; 14) keep caps on all products; 15) be prepared to handle accidents. (Only five are needed.)

CHAPTER 5

1. How can an understanding of anatomy and physiology help you become a better nail technician?

    An understanding of anatomy and physiology can help you become a better nail technician because it will give you a scientific background for many of the nail services you provide. It will help you decide which services are better for clients' nail or skin conditions and how to adjust and control the service for best results.

2. What is the purpose of cells within the human body?

    Cells are the basic functional units of all living things. Cells carry on all life processes and reproduce new cells, enabling the body to replace worn or injured tissues.

3. What is cell metabolism?

    Cell metabolism is a complex chemical process in which cells are nourished and supplied with the elements necessary to carry on their many activities.

4. Name the five types of body tissues and explain the function of each.

    Five types of body tissues are: 1) connective tissue, which supports, protects, and binds the body tissues together; 2) muscular tissue, which contracts and moves various parts of the body; 3) nerve tissue, which carries messages to and from the brain and coordinates all body functions; 4) epithelial tissue, which is a protective covering on body surfaces; 5) liquid tissue, which carries food, wastes, and hormones by means of blood and lymph.

5. What are the five most important organs of the body? Explain the function of each.

    The five most important organs of the body are: 1) the brain, which controls the body; 2) the lungs, which supply oxygen to the blood; 3) the liver, which removes toxic products of digestion; 4) the kidneys, which excrete water and other waste products; 5) the stomach and intestines, which digest food; 6) the heart, which circulates the blood. (Only five are needed.)

6. List the ten systems that make up the human body. What is the function of each system?

    Ten systems making up the human body are: 1) the integumentary system, which functions as a protective covering and contains sensory receptors; 2) the skeletal system, which serves as a means of support, movement, and protection; 3) the muscular system, which produces all movement of the body; 4) the nervous system, which controls and coordinates the functions of all other body systems; 5) the circulatory system, which supplies blood throughout the body; 6) the endocrine system, which secretes hormones into the bloodstream; 7) the excretory system, which eliminates waste from the body; 8) the respiratory system, which supplies oxygen to the body; 9) the digestive system, which changes food into substances that can be used by the body cells; 10) the reproductive system, which allows humans to reproduce.

7. What are four ways in which muscles are stimulated?

    Muscles are stimulated by: 1) massage; 2) electric current; 3) light rays; 4) heat rays; 5) moist heat; 6) nerve impulses; 7) chemicals. (Only four are needed.)

8. What are four types of muscles that are affected by massage?

    Four types of muscles that are affected by massage are: 1) shoulder and upper arm; 2) forearm; 3) hand; 4) lower leg and foot.

9. What are the three divisions of the nervous system? What is the function of each division?

    Three divisions of the nervous system and their functions are: 1) the central nervous system, which controls the voluntary actions of the five senses; 2) the peripheral nervous system, which carries messages to and from the central nervous system; 3) the autonomic nervous system, which regulates the activities of smooth muscles, glands, blood vessels, and the heart.

10. What are the chief functions of the blood?

    The chief functions of the blood are: to carry water, oxygen, food, and secretions to cells; to carry away carbon dioxide and waste products; to help equalize body temperature; to aid in protecting the body from harmful bacteria and infection; and to clot, preventing the loss of blood.

CHAPTER 6

1. What are the three main parts that make up the nail?

    Three parts making up the nail are: 1) nail body (plate); 2) nail root; 3) free edge.

2. Define nail disorder.

   A nail disorder is a condition caused by injury to the nail, disease, or an imbalance in the body.

3. What is the golden rule for dealing with nail disorders?

   The golden rule states that if the nail or skin to be worked on is infected, inflamed, broken, or swollen, a nail technician should refer the client to a doctor.

4. List five nail disorders that can be serviced by a nail technician.

   Five nail disorders that can be serviced by a nail technician are: 1) hangnails; 2) discolored nails; 3) eggshell nails; 4) furrows; 5) leuconychia; 6) onychatrophia or atrophy; 7) onychauxis; 8) onychophagy; 9) onychorrhexis; 10) ptergium; 11) saleronychia. (Only five are needed.)

5. List five nail disorders that cannot be serviced by a nail technician.

   Five nail disorders that cannot be serviced by a nail technician are: 1) mold; 2) onychia; 3) onychogryposis; 4) onycholysis; 5) onychoptosis; 6) paronychia; 7) pyrogenic granuloma. (Only five are needed.)

CHAPTER 7

1. What are the characteristics of healthy skin?

   Healthy skin is characterized by being slightly moist and acid, soft, and flexible. Healthy skin also has elasticity, a smooth, fine-grained texture, and is free of blemishes and diseases.

2. What are five functions of the skin?

   Five functions of the skin are: 1) protection; 2) prevention of fluid loss; 3) response to external stimulus; 4) heat regulation; 5) secretion; 6) excretion; 7) absorption; 8) respiration. (Only five are needed.)

3. Describe the epidermis and dermis.

   The epidermis is the outermost protective covering of the skin. It contains no blood vessels, but does contain many small nerve layers. The dermis is the deep layer of the skin. It contains blood vessels, lymph vessels, nerves, sweat glands, and oil glands in an elastic network made up of collagen.

4. How is skin nourished?

   The skin is nourished by blood and lymph.

5. What are the functions of sweat glands?

   The functions of sweat glands are to regulate body temperature and eliminate waste products through perspiration.

6. Name five types of lesions.

   Five types of lesions are: 1) bulla; 2) crust; 3) cyst; 4) excoriation; 5) fissure; 6) macule; 7) papule; 8) pustule; 9) scales; 10) scars; 11) stain; 12) tubercule; 13) tumor; 14) nodules; 15) ulcers; 16) vesicles; 17) wheals. (Only five are needed.)

7. What are the characteristics of eczema and psoriasis?

   Eczema is characterized by itching, burning, and the formation of scales and oozing blisters. Psoriasis is characterized by a chronic inflammation with round, dry patches covered with coarse silvery scales.

CHAPTER 8

1. What is the purpose of a client consultation?

   The purpose of a client consultation is to discuss the client's general health, the health of his or her nails and skin, and the client's lifestyle in order to select the most appropriate nail service.

2. What are the characteristics of healthy nails?

   Healthy nails are not inflamed, infected, swollen, or broken.

3. How would your services differ for a runner or a guitar player?

   A guitar player may need short nails on the left hand and longer nails on the right. He or she will also need calluses on the fingertips of the left hand. A runner may have calluses on the feet that protect feet while running.

4. Under what circumstances would you refer a client to a physician?

   If an infection, swelling, broken skin, or an inflammation is evident, one should refer a client to a physician.

5. What are the three types of information on the client health/record card?

   The general information asks for the client's name, address, telephone number, and best appointment hours. The client profile asks for information about the type of work and leisure activities the client participates in. The medical record asks for information about the client's general health. This information will help you determine whether it is safe to perform hand and foot massage on the client.

CHAPTER 9

1. When you give a manicure, you need equipment, implements, materials, and nail cosmetics. Give three examples of these manicuring supplies.

    Three examples of equipment used in nail technology are: 1) manicure table with an adjustable lamp; 2) client's chair and nail technician's chair or stool; 3) fingerbowl; 4) wet sanitizer; 5) client's cushion; 6) sanitized cotton container; 7) supply tray; 8) electric nail dryer. (Only three are needed.)
    Materials needed for a manicure include: 1) disposable towels or terry towels; 2) cotton or cotton balls; 3) plastic bags; 4) 70% ethyl alcohol; 5) powder alum or styptic powder. (Only three are needed.)
    Nail cosmetics include: 1) polish remover; 2) cuticle cream; 3) cuticle oil; 4) cuticle solvent; 5) nail bleach; 6) nail whitener; 7) dry nail polish; 8) colored polish; 9) liquid enamel or lacquer; 10) base coat; 11) nail strengthener; 12) top coat or sealer; 13) liquid nail dry; 14) hand cream or lotion. (Only three are needed.)

2. What are two reasons for having a manicuring table that is sanitary and properly equipped?

    Two reasons for having a manicuring table that is sanitary and properly equipped are: 1) anything needed during a service will be at your fingertips; 2) having an orderly table will give you and your client confidence during the manicure.

3. Describe the four basic nail shapes.

    Four basic nail shapes are: 1) rectangular or square; 2) round; 3) oval; 4) pointed.

4. List the six steps in the water manicure pre-service.

    The six steps in the water manicure pre-service are: 1) pre-service sanitation procedure; 2) set up standard manicuring table; 3) greet client; 4) have client wash hands with an antibacterial soap; 5) do client consultation; 6) begin working with the hand that is not the client's favored hand.

5. Briefly describe the water manicure procedure.

    The water manicure procedure is as follows: 1) remove polish; 2) shape nails; 3) soften cuticles; 4) clean nails; 5) dry hand; 6) apply cuticle remover; 7) loosen cuticles; 8) nip cuticles; 9) clean under free edge; 10) repeat steps 4–9 on other hand; 11) bleach nails (optional); 12) buff with chamois buffer (optional); 13) apply cuticle oil; 14) bevel nails; 15) apply hand lotion and massage hand and arm; 16) remove traces of oil; 17) choose color; 18) apply polish.

6. Name the five types of polish applications.

    Five types of polish applications are: 1) full coverage; 2) free edge; 3) hairline tip; 4) half moon or lunula; 5) slimline or free walls.

7. List the five steps in the water manicure post-service.

    The five steps in the water manicure post-service are: 1) make another appointment; 2) sell retail products; 3) clean up around your table; 4) discard used materials; 5) sanitize table and implements.

8. List the four steps in the French manicure procedure.

    Four steps in the French manicure are: 1) apply base coat; 2) apply white polish; 3) apply sheer pink, natural, or peach polish; 4) apply top coat.

9. What are the three benefits of the reconditioning hot oil manicure? How often should clients receive a reconditioning hot oil manicure?

    Three benefits of the reconditioning hot oil manicure are: 1) it is recommended for clients with ridges and brittle nails; 2) it is also recommended for clients with dry cuticles; 3) it improves the hands by leaving the skin soft and adding moisture to hands and nails. A reconditioning manicure is recommended once a week.

10. What type of polish application is included in a man's manicure?

    A man's manicure is the same as a woman's except that a colored polish is not used in a man's manicure.

11. Name five hand massage techniques and five arm massage techniques.

    Five hand massage techniques are: 1) relaxer movement; 2) joint movement on fingers; 3) circular movement in palm; 4) circular movement on wrist; 5) circular movement on back of hand and fingers. Five arm massage techniques are: 1) distribute cream or lotion; 2) effleurage on arms; 3) wringing movements on arm-friction massage movement; 4) kneading movement on arm; 5) rotation of elbow-friction massage movement.

12. What are two safety cautions for hand and arm massage?

    Two safety cautions for hand and arm massage are: 1) avoid vigorous joint massage if your client has arthritis; 2) do not massage if your client has high blood pressure, a heart condition, or has had a stroke.

CHAPTER 10

1. Name five pedicure supplies.

   Five pedicure supplies are: 1) pedicure station; 2) pedicure stool and footrest; 3) client's chair; 4) rinse and soap baths; 5) toe separators; 6) foot file; 7) toenail clippers; 8) antiseptic fungal foot spray; 9) antibacterial soap; 10) foot lotion; 11) foot powder; 12) pedicure slippers. (Only five are needed.)

2. List the eight steps in the pedicure pre-service.

   The steps in the pedicure pre-service include: 1) pre-service sanitation procedure; 2) setting up the pedicure station; 3) spread one terry cloth towel on the floor in front of the client's chair, spread another over the stool to dry feet; 4) place pedicuring materials on standard manicuring table; 5) set up standard manicuring table in pedicure station; 6) both basins should be filled with warm water and antibacterial soap in one and antiseptic in the other; 7) greet client; 8) complete client consultation.

3. Briefly describe the pedicure procedure.

   The pedicure procedure includes: 1) removing shoes and socks; 2) spraying feet; 3) soaking feet; 4) rinsing feet; 5) drying feet; 6) removing polish; 7) clipping nails; 8) inserting toe separators; 9) filing nails; 10) using foot file to remove dry skin and callus growths; 11) rinsing the foot; 12) repeating steps 7–11 on other foot; 13) brushing nails; 14) applying cuticle solvent; 15) pushing back the cuticle; 16) brushing the foot; 17) applying lotion; 18) massaging foot; 19) proceed with steps 13–19 on other foot; 20) remove traces of lotion; 21) apply polish; 22) powder feet.

4. Describe the proper technique to use in filing toenails.

   Toenails are filed straight across, rounded slightly at the corners to conform to the shape of the toes. Do not file into the corners of nails. Rough edges are to be smoothed with the fine side of the emery board.

5. List the six steps in the pedicure post-service.

   Post service pedicure steps include: scheduling another appointment; advising client about foot care; selling retail products; cleaning pedicure area; discarding used materials; sanitizing table and implements.

6. Name six foot massage techniques.

   Six foot massage techniques include: 1) relaxer movement to the joints of the foot; 2) effleurage on the top of the foot; 3) effleurage on heel; 4) effleurage movement on toes; 5) joint movement for toes; 6) thumb impression-friction movement; 7) metatarsal scissors; 8) fist twist compression; 9) effleurage on instep; 10) percussion or tapotement movement. (Only six are needed.)

7. What is a safety caution for pedicuring?

   A safety caution for a pedicure is to ask clients if they are being treated for high blood perssure, heart condition, or diabetes.

CHAPTER 11

1. List four supplies, in addition to your basic manicuring table, that you need for nail tip application.

   Four supplies needed for nail tip application, in addition to the basic manicuring table, are: 1) abrasive; 2) a buffer block; 3) nail adhesive; 4) nail tips.

2. Name two types of nail tips.

   Two types of nail tips are plastic, nylon, and acetate. (Only two are needed.)

3. What portion of the natural nail plate should be covered by a nail tip?

   Nail tips should cover no more than one-half the natural nail plate.

4. What type of tip application is considered a temporary service? Why?

   Applying a tip without an overlay, such as a fabric wrap or acrylic nail, is considered a temporary service because a tip without such a service is very weak.

5. Briefly describe the procedure for nail tip application.

   The procedure for nail tip application is as follows: 1) remove all polish; 2) push back cuticle; 3) buff nail to remove shine; 4) clean nails; 5) size tips; 6) apply nail antiseptic; 7) apply adhesive; 8) slide on tips; 9) apply adhesive bead to seam; 10) trim nail tip; 11) blend tip into natural nail; 12) buff tip for perfect blend; 13) shape nail; 14) proceed with desired service.

6. Describe the proper maintenance of nail tips.

   The proper maintenance for nail tips is to follow with weekly or biweekly manicures for regluing and rebuffing. Non-acetone polish remover should be used because acetone dissolves the tips.

7. Describe the procedure for the removal of tips.

   The procedure for removing tips is as follows: 1) complete nail tip application pre-service procedure; 2) soak nails; 3) slide off tip; 4) buff nail; 5) condition cuticle and surrounding skin; 6) proceed with desired service; 7) complete nail tip application post-service if no further service is performed.

CHAPTER 12

1. List four kinds of nail wraps.

   Four kinds of nail wraps are 1) silk; 2) linen; 3) fiberglass; 4) paper wraps.

2. Explain the benefits of using silk, linen, fiberglass, and paper wraps.

   The benefits for silk, linen, fiberglass, and paper wraps are as follows: 1) silk wraps are strong, lightweight, and smooth when applied to nails; 2) linen is thicker than silk or fiberglass; linen is strong and lasts a long time; 3) fiberglass has a loose weave, which makes for easy penetration of the adhesive; it's especially strong and durable; 4) paper wraps are temporary.

3. Describe the procedure for fabric wrap application.

   The procedure for fabric wrap application is as follows: 1) remove old polish; 2) clean nails; 3) push cuticle back; 4) buff nail to remove shine; 5) apply nail antiseptic; 6) apply glue; 7) cut fabric; 8) apply fabric adhesives; 9) apply fabric; 10) trim fabric; 11) apply fabric adhesive; 12) apply fabric adhesive dryer; 13) apply second coat of adhesive; 14) apply second coat of adhesive dryer; 15) shape and refine nails; 16) buff nails; 17) apply hand lotion; 18) remove traces of oil; 19) apply polish.

4. Explain how a fabric wrap is used as a crack repair.

   A fabric wrap is used as a crack repair by cutting a repair patch to completely cover the crack or break.

5. Describe how to remove fabric wraps and what to avoid.

   The fabric wrap removal procedure is as follows: 1) complete nail wrap pre-service; 2) soak nails; 3) slide off softened wraps; 4) buff nails; 5) condition cuticles. Avoid damaging the nail plate when removing fabric wraps.

6. Describe the purpose of paper wraps and explain why they are not recommended for very long nails.

   The purpose of paper wraps is to provide a temporary method of strengthening the nail. Paper wraps are not recommended for very long nails because they do not provide the strength that long nails require.

7. List the materials used for paper wraps.

   The materials used in paper wraps are mending tissues, mending liquid, and ridge fillers.

8. Outline the procedure used in paper wraps.

   The procedure used in paper wraps is as follows: 1) complete nail wrap pre-service; 2) remove old nail polish; 3) clean nails; 4) push back cuticles; 5) buff nails to remove shine; 6) apply nail antiseptic; 7) tear mending tissue; 8) apply mending liquid to tissue; 9) apply paper wrap; 10) smooth the wrap; 11) cut tissue; 12) apply mending liquid under free edge; 13) smooth wrap; 14) refine nail; 15) apply mending liquid; 16) apply ridge filler; 17) apply polish; 18) complete nail wrap post-service.

9. Define liquid nail wrap and describe its purpose.

   Liquid nail wrap is a polish made of tiny fibers designed to strengthen and preserve the natural nail as it grows. After it has been brushed on the nail in several directions and allowed to harden, it creates a network that protects the nail.

CHAPTER 13

1. List the supplies needed for acrylic nail application.

   The supplies needed for acrylic nail application are: acrylic liquid, acrylic powder, primer, abrasive, small containers for liquid and powder acrylic, nail forms, sable brush, safety glasses, and plastic gloves.

2. Briefly describe the chemistry of acrylic nails.

   The chemistry of acrylic nails is broken down into three basic ingredients. A monomer is made up of many small molecules that aren't attached to each other. Liquid acrylic is a monomer. A polymer is made up of molecules that are attached to each other in long chains, usually forming something hard. Finished acrylic nails are polymers. A catalyst speeds up the hardening process. Powdered acrylic is a combination of ground up polymer and a catalyst. Polymerization is the process of forming the nail.

3. Describe the procedure for the application of acrylic nails over forms.

    The procedure for applying acrylic nails over forms is as follows: 1) complete acrylic application pre-service; 2) remove polish; 3) clean nails; 4) push back cuticle; 5) buff nail to remove shine; 6) apply nail antiseptic; 7) position nail form; 8) apply primer; 9) prepare acrylic liquid and powder; 10) dip brush into liquid; 11) form acrylic ball; 12) place ball of acrylic on free edge; 13) shape free edge; 14) place second ball of acrylic; 15) shape second ball of acrylic; 16) apply acrylic beads; 17) apply acrylic to remaining nails; 18) shape nails; 19) buff nail; 20) apply cuticle oil; 21) apply hand cream and massage hand and arm; 22) clean nails; 23) apply polish.

4. Describe the safety precautions for applying primer.

    The safety precautions for applying primer are: never use primer without plastic gloves and safety glasses; offer a pair of safety glasses to the client. Check primer on a regular basis to make sure it isn't contaminated with bacteria.

5. Describe the procedure for applying acrylic nails over tips.

    The procedure for applying acrylic nails over tips is as follows: 1) complete acrylic application pre-service; 2) remove polish; 3) clean nails; 4) push back cuticle; 5) buff nail to remove shine; 6) apply nail antiseptic; 7) apply tips; 8) apply primer; 9) prepare acrylic liquid and powder; 10) dip brush into liquid; 11) form acrylic ball; 12) place ball of acrylic on free edge; 13) shape free edge; 14) place second ball of acrylic; 15) shape second ball of acrylic; 16) apply acrylic beads; 17) shape and refine nail; 18) buff nail; 19) apply cuticle oil; 20) apply hand cream and massage hand and arm; 21) clean nails; 22) apply polish; 23) do standard post-service procedure.

6. How does the procedure for acrylic nail application over bitten nails differ from other acrylic nail procedures?

    The procedure for acrylic nail application over bitten nails requires you to create a portion of the nail plate before applying the nail form.

7. Describe the two basic types of maintenance for acrylic nails.

    The two basic types of maintenance for acrylic nails are fill-in and crack repair. Fill-in allows nails to look natural and even while growing out. Crack repair is the addition of extra acrylic to fill the crack in an acrylic nail and reinforce the rest of the nail.

8. Describe the proper procedure for acrylic removal.

   The proper procedure for acrylic removal is as follows: 1) fill bowl with acetone; 2) soak fingertips; 3) remove acrylic with orangewood stick; 4) buff nails; 5) condition cuticle.

9. Explain how the application of odorless acrylics differs from the application of traditional acrylics.

   The application of odorless acrylics is different from the application of traditional acrylics because odorless acrylics do not smell as strongly, they're wetter than traditional acrylics, and they require less shaping. When nails are dry, the surface has a tacky, gummy residue that rolls off as you refine the nails.

CHAPTER 14

1. Describe the two basic types of gel.

   The two basic types of gel are: 1) light-cured gels, which harden when exposed to a special light source such as an ultraviolet light or halogen light; 2) no-light gels, which harden when a gel activator is sprayed or brushed on, or when they are soaked in water.

2. List the supplies needed for light-gel application.

   The supplies needed for light-gel application are: light-cured gel, curing light, brush, nail forms, primer (if recommended by gel manufacturer), block buffer, nail tips, adhesive, and nail art supplies.

3. Describe the proper procedure and precautions for light-cured gel application.

   The proper procedure for light-cured gel is as follows: 1) remove polish; 2) clean nails; 3) push back cuticles; 4) buff nails to remove shine; 5) apply nail antiseptic; 6) apply tips if desired; 7) apply primer if recommended; 8) apply gel; 9) cure gel; 10) repeat steps 8 and 9 on the other hand; 11) apply second coat of gel to the first hand; 12) cure gel; 13) repeat steps 11 and 12 on other hand; 14) repeat steps 11–13; 15) clean nails; 16) apply cuticle oil; 17) apply hand cream and massage hand and arm; 18) clean nails; 19) apply polish. The safety caution for light-cured gel application is that inadequately shielded ultraviolet lamps can damage skin and eyes.

4. Describe the proper procedure and precautions for light-gel application over forms.

   The proper procedure for light-cured gel application over forms is: 1) complete gel application pre-service; 2) apply nail forms; 3) apply gel to natural nail; 4) cure gel; 5) create free edge; 6) cure gel; 7) apply gel to entire nail; 8) cure gel; 9) remove forms; 10) shape free edge; 11) apply gel to entire nail without form; 12) cure gel; 13) remove residue; 14) apply cuticle oil; 15) apply hand cream and massage hand and arm; 16) clean nails; 17) apply polish; 18) complete gel application post-service.

5. Describe no-light gel application.

   No-light gel application includes: 1) gel application pre-service; 2) remove polish; 3) clean nails; 4) push back cuticles; 5) buff nails to remove shine; 6) apply nail antiseptic; 7) apply tips if desired; 8) apply gel; 9) cure gel with activator or water; 10) repeat steps 8 and 9 on the other hand; 11) apply second coat of gel and cure if necessary; 12) shape and refine nails; 13) buff nails to remove shine; 14) apply cuticle oil; 15) apply hand cream and massage hand and arm; 16) clean nails; 17) apply polish; 18) do gel application post-service.

6. Why should you develop nail art skills?

   You should develop nail art skills because nail art is a creative part of a nail technician's job. It turns nails into small canvasses on which you can paint pictures, designs, and collages with tiny gems, foils, or tapes.

CHAPTER 15

1. What are the advantages and disadvantages of working in a full-service salon?

   The advantages of working in a full-service salon are that you automatically get all of the nail business, your services make it convenient for clients to have their nails done while they're there for hair-care or skin-care services. You can also attract clients by offering special rates for nail care while they are having other services performed. Disadvantages of working in a full-service salon include not having other nail technicians to share ideas and experiences with. You may also be limited in the variety of services that you're allowed to perform if you work in a traditional salon. There also won't be someone to fill in for you when you're sick or on vacation.

2. What are the advantages and disadvantages of working in a nails-only salon?

   Advantages of working in a nails-only salon include having the opportunity to share ideas and experiences with other nail technicians and serving their clients when they are sick or on vacation. Disadvantages include competition for clients in a salon with many nail technicians.

3. What are ten questions that will help you determine if a salon is right for you?

   Ten questions that will help you determine if the salon is right for you are: 1) Will the salon provide additional training? 2) Will the salon help you build clientele? 3) Will you be considered an employee, or an independent contractor who rents a booth? 4) If you are an employee, how will the salon pay you? 5) Will the salon provide nail care products or will you have to bring your own? 6) Does the salon offer benefits? 7) Are there fixed or flexible working hours? 8) What is the dress code? 9) Does the salon close for regular vacation periods or does each employee take a separate vacation? 10) What is the salon's reputation? 11) Does the salon have safe working conditions? (Only ten are needed.)

4. What are eight questions that will help you determine if a salon has safe working conditions?

   Eight questions that will help you determine if a salon has safe working conditions are: 1) Does it have proper ventilation? 2) Does it provide separate refrigerators for food and nail product storage? 3) Are MSDS sheets on display or within easy access to employees? 4) Are work stations well-equipped and clean? 5) Are nail technicians required to wear dust masks? 6) Are nail technicians required to wear safety glasses? 7) Are aerosol cans used or are safer application methods used? 8) Are salon workers ready for emergencies?

5. Explain the difference between income and expenses and give two examples of each.

   Income is the money you make. It includes salary, commission from services, commission from retail product sales, and tips. (Only two are needed.) Expenses are what you spend. They include equipment, supplies, books explaining techniques, comfortable shoes, uniforms, and tuition for courses on nail techniques. (Only two are needed.)

6. List four practical uses for business records that are required by local, state, and federal laws.

   Four practical uses for business records required by local, state, and federal laws are: 1) determining income, profits, losses, or expenses; 2) providing the value of your clientele, or the salon's worth to prospective buyers; 3) getting a bank loan; 4) computing income tax, social security, unemployment, and disability insurance.

7. List five types of information that a salon can gather by keeping accurate business records.

    Five types of information that can be gathered by keeping accurate records are: 1) profit and loss comparisons with other weeks, months, or years; 2) changes in demands for services; 3) inventory; 4) net income; 5) material and supply levels.

8. Discuss the advantages of keeping proper service, inventory, and personal appointment records.

    The advantages of keeping proper service, inventory, and personal appointment records are that service records can help another nail technician fill in for a client's usual technician; service records can record client's personal information; inventory records should be kept for use and retail value; personal records will help you arrange your work time for the client's convenience.

9. List nine guidelines that should be followed in booking appointments.

    Nine guidelines that should be followed in booking appointments are: 1) keep a supply of appointment books, pencils, erasers, pens, a calendar, and message pad within reach; 2) be prompt; 3) identify yourself and the salon when answering the phone; 4) be pleasant; 5) take the client's home phone number, type of service to be performed, and date and time of appointment when scheduling appointments; 6) speak clearly; 7) be tactful and courteous when speaking; 8) if you have appointments made in advance, call the night before to remind clients; 9) at the end of the appointment, ask clients if they wish to reschedule.

CHAPTER 16

1. What are the five basic steps in selling.

    Five basic steps in selling are: 1) knowing your products and services; 2) knowing the needs and wants of your clients; 3) presenting your products and services; 4) answering your client's questions and objections properly; 5) close the sale.

2. Describe the difference between product features and benefits.

    A product's feature is a specific fact about it (or a service) that describes it. The benefits of a product or service are what it will do for your client or how it will fulfill your clients wants and needs.

3. Choose one of the nail services you have learned about in this book. Describe two features and two benefits of that service.

   Two features of colored gel nails over tips include the fact that they are lightweight and come in a variety of colors. Two benefits of colored gel nails over tips are long, beautiful nails that will save you both time and money. (Check with your instructor for other correct answers.)

4. What are three questions you should try to answer as you determine your client's needs and wants?

   Three questions that you should try to answer as you determine your client's needs and wants are: 1) Does your client have special nail problems? 2) What is your client's lifestyle? 3) Is your client preparing for a special occasion?

5. Explain how you can sell while you work.

   You can sell while you work by displaying a list of your services and displaying a list of your products. Tell clients what you are doing, what products you are using, and why.

6. List and describe the three steps in closing a sale.

   Three steps in closing a sale are: 1) suggestion selling, which occurs when you suggest services or products for your client to buy; 2) wrap up, which can be used to ask if you can wrap up a product and ask how the client will be paying for the product; 3) schedule another appointment for maintenance of the service you have performed.

Glossary/Index

Note: Boldface entries are definitions.

Abductor hallucis (ab-DUK-tohr ha-LU-sis), **is a muscle of the foot,** 51
Abductors (ab-DUK-tohrs), **separate the fingers,** 50
Acquired immune deficiency syndrome (AIDS), is a disease caused by the HIV virus, 17-18
Acquired immunity, 20
Acrylic (a-KRYL-uk) **nails, are made by combining a liquid acrylic product with a powdered acrylic product,** 152
  application,
    post-service, 157-158
    pre-service, 153
    procedure, 153-157
  maintenance, 162-165
  odorless, 166
  over,
    bitten nails, 160-162
    tips/natural nails, 158-160
  removal, 165
  supplies for, 152-153
Adductors (a-DUK-tohrs), **draw the fingers together,** 50
Adipose (AD-i-pohs), **a fatty tissue that is part of the subcutaneous tissue,** 76
Advertising, 189
Afferent (AF-fer-ent) **nerves, carry impulses or messages from sense organs to the brain,** 53
Agnails, also known as hangnails, is a common condition in which the cuticle around the nail splits, 66
AIDS. *See* acquired immune deficiency syndrome (AIDS), 17-18
Air brush, nail art and, 180
Albinism (AL-bi-niz-em), **is a congenital absence of melanin pigment in the body, including the skin, hair, and eyes,** 81
Alcohol
  manicure and, 97
  sanitation with, 28
Alum, manicure and, 97
Anabolism (ah-NAB-o-liz-em), **is the process of building up larger molecules from smaller ones,** 42
Anterior tibial (TIB-ee-al) **artery, goes to the foot and becomes the dorsalis pedis,** 58
Antibacterial soap, 97
Antiseptic (an-ti-SEP-tik), **is usually a liquid that may kill or retard the growth of bacteria,** 25
Appearance, professional, 12-13
Appointments, booking, 187-188, 195
Arm
  massage, 117-119
  upper, muscles of, 49
Arrectores pili (a-REK-tohr PIGH-ligh), **muscles that are attached to the hair follicles and can cause goose bumps,** 76
Arteries, are thick-walled muscular and elastic tubes that carry oxygen-filled blood from the heart to the capillaries throughout the body, 56

Athlete's foot, also known as tinea pedis (TIN-ee-ah PEH-dus) **or ringworm of the foot, is a fungus infection of the foot,** 81
Atria, upper chambers of the heart, 56
Atrium (AY-tree-um), **the upper, thin-walled chambers of the heart,** 56
Auricle (OR-ik-kel), **upper chambers of the heart,** 56
Autoclave, a machine that uses steam pressure to sanitize, 25
Autonomic (aw-toh-NAHM-ik) **nervous system, is the portion of the nervous system that functions without conscious effort and regulates the activities of the smooth muscles, glands, blood vessels, and heart,** 52
Axon (AK-son), **sends messages to other neurons, glands, or muscles,** 53

Bacilli (bah-SIL-i), **are the most common bacteria. They are rod-shaped and produce such diseases as tetanus, influenza, typhoid, tuberculosis, and diphtheria,** 16
Bacteria (bak-TEER-i-ah), **are one-celled vegetable microorganisms,** 15
  growth/reproduction of, 17
  movement of, 17
  pathogenic, classification of, 16
  types of, 15-16
Bags, plastic, manicure and, 97
Ball-and-socket joint, one bone is rounded and fits into the socket, or hollow part, of another bone, 45
Base coat, is colorless and is applied to the natural nail before the application of colored polish, 99
Biceps, is the muscle on the front of the upper arm that lifts the forearm, flexes the elbow, and turns the palm up, 49
Birthmark, or nevus (NEE-vus) **is a malformation of the skin due to abnormal pigmentation or dilated capillaries,** 82
Blood
  is a nutritive fluid that moves throughout the circulatory system, 56
  circulation of, 56
  composition of, 57
  function of, 57
  platelets (PLAY-tel-lets), **are much smaller than the red blood cells; they help blood to clot,** 57
  supply to,
    arm and hand, 57-58
    lower leg and foot, 58
  vascular system, consists of the heart and blood vessels for the circulation of blood, 55
  vessels are tubelike in construction. They transport blood to and from the heart and to various parts of the body, 56
Boiling, sanitation and, 25
Bones
  arm/hand, 45-46
  leg/foot, 46-47
  structure of, 45
Brain
  controls the body, 43
  nervous system and, 52-53

Bruised nails, is a condition in which a clot of blood forms under the nail, 65
Bulla (BYOO-lah), is a blister containing watery fluid, 79
Business records, 186

Cabinet sanitizer, is an airtight cabinet in which formaldehyde tablets are placed. These will produce an active fumigant, 26
Calcaneous (kal-KAY-nee-us) bone, or heel, is considered to be part of the ankle, 46
Callus, or keratoma, is an acquired superficial, round and thickened patch of epidermis due to pressure or friction on the hands and feet, 82
Capillaries, are tiny, thin-walled blood vessels that connect the smaller arteries to the veins. Through their walls, the tissues receive nourishment and eliminate waste products, 56
Cardiac (CAR-dee-ak) muscle, is heart muscle, which is not found anywhere else in the body, 48
Carpus (KAHR-pus), or wrist, is a flexible joint composed of eight small, irregular bones held together by ligaments, 46
Cartilage (CAR-tih-ledg), is a tough elastic substance similar to bone but it has no mineral content, 45
Catabolism (kah-TAB-o-liz-em), is the breaking down of larger substances or molecules into smaller ones, 43
Cell
  growth, 42
  membrane, encloses the cytoplasm, 41
  metabolism, 42-43
Central nervous system, consists of the brain and spinal cord, 52
Centrosome (SEN-tro-sohm), is a small round body in the cytoplasm and affects the reproduction of the cell, 41
Cerebro-spinal (ser-EE-broh SPEYE-nahl), system consists of the brain and spinal cord, 52
Chamois (SHAM-ee) buffer, manicure and, 95-96
Chemicals
  commonly used, 33
  sanitizing agents, 27-28
  solutions, agents for making, 26-27
Chlosama (kloh-AZ-mah), are brown spots on the skin, especially the face and hands. They are also called "liver spots" or "moth patches," 82
Cilia (SIL-ee-a), hairlike projections that move in a whiplike motion, 17
Circulatory (SUR-kyoo-lah-tohr-ee) system
  controls the steady circulation of the blood through the body by means of the heart and blood vessels, 55
  supplies blood throughout the body, 44
Clavicle (KLAV-i-kul), is also known as the collar bone, 45
Client
  conduct toward, 7-8
  health/record card of, 86-87, 89
  protecting, 36-38
  selling products to, 191-195
  service record, 88
Clippers, fingernail, 96
Cocci (KOK-si), round, pus-producing bacteria, 16
Colored polish, is used to add color and gloss to the nail, 98
Common peroneal (per-oh-NEE-al) nerve, a division of the sciatica nerve, is located behind the knee and has two parts, 54
Connective tissue, serves to support, protect, and bind together tissues of the body, 43
Corium, is the deep layer of the skin and is also called the "true skin," 76

Cotton
  balls, manicure and, 97
  container for, manicure and, 93
Cuticle (KYOO-ti-kel), is the overlapping skin around the nail, 64
  cream, 98
  nipper, manicure and, 95
  oil, 98
  remover, 98
  solvent, 98
Cutis, is the deep layer of the skin and is also called the "true skin," 76
Cyst (SIST), is a semisolid or fluid lump above and below the skin surface, 79
Cytoplasm (SEYE-toh-plaz-em), is found outside the nucleus and contains food materials necessary for the growth, reproduction, and self-repair of the cell, 41

Decomposing (de-kom-POH-zing), breaking down of matter, 15
Deep peroneal nerve, passes down the back of the leg, 54
Deltoid (DEL-toid), is a large, thick triangular muscle that covers the shoulder and lifts and turns the arm, 49
Dendrites (DEN-dreytes), receive messages from other neurons, 53
Derma, is the deep layer of the skin and is also called the "true skin," 76
Dermatology (dere-mah-TOL-o-jee), the study of healthy skin and skin disorders, 73
Dermis, is the deep layer of the skin and is also called the "true skin," 76
Diaphragm, is a muscular partition that controls breathing, and separates the chest from the abdominal region, 60
Digestion, is the process of converting food into a form that can be used by the body, 60
Digestive enzymes, are chemicals that change certain kinds of food into a form capable of being used by the body, 60
Digestive system
  changes food into soluble form, suitable for use by the cells of the body, 60
  changes food into substances that can be used by the body, 44
Digital (DIJ-it-al nerve), and its branches supply all fingers of the hand, 54
Diplococci (deye-ploh-KOK-si), grow in pairs and cause pneumonia, 16
Discolored nails, is a condition in which the nails turn a variety of colors including yellow, blue, blue-grey, green, red, and purple, 65
Disinfectant (dis-in-FEK-tant), is stronger than an antiseptic. It destroys most bacteria, 25
  approved, 28
Dorsal (DOOR-sal) nerve, supplies impulses to the top of the foot, 54
Dorsalis pedis artery, supplies blood to the foot, 58
Dry nail polish, or pumice powder is used with the chamois buffer to add shine to the nail, 98
  heat, sanitation and, 25
  sanitizer, is an airtight cabinet in which formaldehyde tablets are placed. These will produce an active fumigant, 26
Dryer, nail, electric, 94

Eczema (EK-se-mah), is a chronic, long-lasting disorder of unknown cause, 80
Efferent (EF-fer-ent) nerves, carry impulses from the brain to the muscles, 53

Eggshell nails, are thin, white, and curved over the free edge. The condition is caused by improper diet, internal disease, medication, or nervous disorders, 65
Elastic tissue, in the papillary layer of the dermis gives the skin its ability to return to its original shape after it has been stretched, 78
Electric manicure, 115-116
Emery board, manicure and, 95
Employers, coworkers and, 9
Endocrine (EN-doh-krin)
   glands, secrete hormones, 59
   system, is made up of ductless glands that secrete hormones into the bloodstream, 44, 59
Epidermis (ep-i-DUR-mis), also called the cuticle or scarf skin, is the outermost protection covering the skin, 75
Epithelial (ep-i-THE-le-al) tissue, is a protective covering on body surfaces, such as the skin, mucous membranes, linings of the ear, digestive and respiratory organs, and glands, 43
Eponychium (ep-o-NIK-ee-um), is the thin line of skin at the base of the nail that extends from the nail wall and nail plate, 64
Esophagus (i-SOF-a-gus), 60
Ethics
   toward clients, 10
   toward employer/coworkers, 11-12
Ethyl alcohol, manicure and, 97
Excoriation (ed-skohr-i-AY-shun), is a sore or abrasion caused by scratching or scraping, 79
Excretory (EK-skre-tohr-ee) system
   eliminates waste from the body, 44
   includes the kidneys, liver, skin, intestines, and lungs, and purifies the body by eliminating waste matter, 59
Exhale, carbon dioxide is expelled, 60
Extensor (eck-STEN-sur),
   digitorum brevis (ek-STEN-sur dij-it-TOHR-um BREV-us), is a muscle of the foot, 51
   digitorum longus (eck-STEN-sur dij-it-TOHR-um LONG-us), bends the foot up and extends the toes, 51
   straightens the wrist, hand, and fingers to form a straight line, 49

Fabric nail wrap
   maintenance, 145-147
   removal, 147
   repairs, 147
Femur (FEE-mur), is a heavy, long bone that forms the leg above the knee, 46
Fibula (FIB-ya-lah), is the smaller of the two bones that form the leg below the knee, 46
Fingerbowl, manicure and, 93
Fingernail clippers, manicure and, 96
Fissure (FISH-ur), is a crack in the skin that penetrates the dermis. Chapped hands or lips are an example of fissure, 79
Flagella (flah-JEL-ah), hairlike projections that move in a whiplike motion, 17
Flexor digitorum brevis (FLEKS-or dij-it-TOHR-um BREV-us), is a muscle of the foot, 51
Flexors (FLEKS-ors), bend to the wrist, draw the hand upward, and close the fingers toward the forearm, 49
Foil, nail art and, 177
Foot
   massage, 127-129
   muscles of, 50-51

Forearm, contains a series of muscles and strong tendons, 49
Formaldehyde strengthener, contains five percent formaldehyde, 99
Formalin (FOHR-mah-lin), is a sanitizing agent used as a disinfectant comprised of formaldehyde gas in water, 27-28
Freckles, or lentigines (len-ti-JEE-neez), are small brown or yellow spots, 82
French manicure, 109
Fumigant (FYUM-i-gant), is a kind of disinfectant and is used with a dry or cabinet sanitizer, 25
Fundus (FUN-dus), a tubelike duct that ends at the skin surface to form a sweat pore, 77
Fungi (FUN-gi), is the general term for vegetable parasites including all types of fungus and mold, 18
Furrows, in nails, also known as corrugations, are long ridges that run either lengthwise or across the nail, 65-66

Gastrocnemius (gas-truc-NEEM-e-us), is attached to the lower rear surface of the heel and pulls the foot down, 51
Gel
   application,
      post-service, 172
      pre-service, 170
      procedure, 170-172
   maintenance, 175
   no-light, application, 174-175
   over, forms, 172-173
   removal, 175
   supplies for, 169-170
Gems, nail art and, 176
General circulation, is the blood circulation from the heart throughout the body and back again to the heart, 56
Gland, is a specialized organ that secretes substances, 59
Gliding joints, two bones glide over each other, 45
Gold, nail art and, 179-180
Golden rule, if the nail or skin to be worked on is infected, broken, or swollen, a nail technician should not service the client, 65, 78

Hand, cream/lotion, soften and smooth the hands, 99
   massage, 116-117
Hangnails, also known as agnails, is a common condition in which the cuticle around the nail splits, 66
Health/record card, client's, 86-87, 89
Heart, circulates the blood, 43
   is a muscular, cone-shaped organ about the size of a closed fist. It is located in the chest cavity, and is enclosed in a membrane, 55
   diagram of, 55
   valves, allow the blood to flow in only one direction, 56
   chambers of, 56
Heat, sanitation and, 25
Herpes simplex, is a skin infection common in dental staff and others involved with care of the mouth, 81
Hinge (HINJ) joints, two or more bones that connect like a door, 45
Hives, are swollen, itchy bumps on the skin that last for several hours, 80
Holly berries, procedure for, 178-179
Homeostasis (ho-me-oh-STAY-sus), is the maintenance of normal, internal, stability in the body, 43
Hormones, chemicals that affect metabolism and other body processes, directly into the bloodstream, 59

Humerus (HYOO-mo-rus), is the uppermost and largest bone of the arm, 45
Hypertrophy (hy-PER-troh-fee), is the overgrowth of nails, 66-67
  definitions pertaining to, 82
Hyponychium (heye-poh-NIK-ee-um), is the part of the skin under the free edge of the nail, 64

Immunity (i-MYOO-ni-tee)
  is the ability of the body to resist disease and destroy microorganisms when they have entered the body, 19
  acquired, 20
  natural, 20
Infection (in-FEK-shun), an area that shows evidence of pus, 65
  immunity to, 19-20
  occurs when body tissue is invaded by disease-causing microorganisms, 19
  prevention of, 21
  salons and, 20-21
Inflammation (in-flam-MAY-shun), an area that is red and sore, 65
Ingrown nails, the nail grows into the sides of the tissue around the nail, 67
Inhale, oxygen is absorbed into the blood, 60
Integumentary (in-TEG-yoo-men-ta-ree) system, is made up of the skin and its various accessory organs, 44
Intestines, digest food, 43
Inventory records, 187

Joints, junctions where bones of the body meet, 45

Keratoma, or callus, is an acquired superficial, round and thickened patch of epidermis due to pressure or friction on the hands and feet, 82
Kidneys, excrete water and other waste products, 43

Lacquer (LAK-er), is used to add color and gloss to the nail, 98
Left
  atrium (AY-tree-um), one of the upper, thin-walled chambers of the heart, 56
  ventricle (VEN-tri-kel), one of the lower, thick-walled chambers of the heart, 56
Leg, lower, muscles of, 50-51
Lentigines (len-ti-JEE-neez), or freckles, are small brown or yellow spots, 82
Lesion (LEE-zhun)
  is a structural change in tissue caused by injury and disease, 79
  skin, is a structural change in tissue caused by injury and disease, 79
Leucoderma (loo-ko-DER-ma), a general term for the abnormal lack of pigmentation, 81
Leuconychia (loo-ko-NIK-ee-ah), is a condition in which white spots appear on the nails, 66
Ligaments (LIG-e-mentz), are bands or sheets of fibrous tissue that support the bones at the joints, 45
Light-cured gel. *See* gel
Liquid
  enamel, is used to add color and gloss to the nail, 98
  nail dry, is used to prevent smudging of the polish, 99
  nail wrap, 149
  tissue, carries food, waste products, and hormones by means of the blood and lymph, 43
Liver, removes toxic products of digestion, 43
Lungs
are spongy tissues composed of microscopic cells that take in air, 60
supply oxygen to the blood, 43
Lymph (LIMF)
  system, consists of lymph glands and vessels through which a colorless fluid called lymph circulates, 55
  is a colorless, watery fluid that is made from the plasma of the blood, 58-59
  vascular system, also called the lymphatic system, acts as an aid to the blood system, and consists of lymph spaces, lymph vessels, and lymph glands, 58
Lymphatic (lim-FAT-ik) system
  acts as an aid to the blood system, and consists of lymph spaces, lymph vessels, and lymph glands, 58
  consists of lymph glands and vessels through which a colorless fluid called lymph circulates, 55

Macule (MAK-ul), is a small, discolored spot or patch on the surface of the skin, 79
Manicure
  alum, 97
  chamois buffer, 95-96
  client's cushion, 93
  cotton balls, 97
  cotton container, sanitized, 93
  cuticle nipper, 95
  electric, 115-116
  emery board, 95
  ethyl alcohol, 97
  fingerbowl, 93
  fingernail clippers, 96
  French, 109
  man's, 111-114
  materials for, 96-97
  nail brush, 95
  nail dryer, electric, 94
  nail file, metal, 94
  orangewood stick, 94
  plastic bags, 97
  reconditioning hot oil, 109-110
    pre-service, 110
    procedure, 110-111
  sanitation, implements and, 96
  spatula, 97
  steel pusher, 94
  styptic powder, 97
  supplies for,
    equipment, 93-94
    implements, 94-96
  supply tray for, 94
  table, 93
    set-up procedure, 100-101
  towels,
    disposable, 97
    terry cloth, 97
  tweezers, 95
  water,
    post-service, 108
    pre-service, 102-103
    procedure, 103-108
Man's manicure, 111-114
Mantle (MAN-tel), also called nail fold, is the deep fold of skin at the base of the nail where the nail root is embedded, 64
Marbled gold, nail art and, 179-180

GLOSSARY/INDEX 221

Massage
  arm, 117-119
  foot, 127-129
  hand, 116-117
  muscles affected by, 49-51
Material Safety Data Sheets (MSDS), contain twelve basic items of information on manufacturers' products, 34-35
Median (MEE-di-an) nerve, is a smaller nerve than the ulnar and radial nerves. With its branches, it supplies the arm and hand, 54
Melanin (MEL-a-nin), skin pigment that determines skin color and protects sensitive skin cells below from the destructive effects of excessive ultraviolet rays from the sun or an ultraviolet lamp, 75
Melanotic sarcoma, is a fatal skin cancer that begins with the growth of a mole, 82
Metabolism (meh-TAB-o-liz-em), is a complex chemical process whereby the body cells are nourished and supplied with the energy needed to carry on their many activities, 42
Metacarpals (met-a-KAHR-puls), the bones of the palm of the hand, are long and slender, 46
Metatarsals (met-ah-TAHR-suls), of the foot are long and slender like the metacarpal bones of the hand, 46
Microorganisms (meye-kroh-OR-gah-niz-ems), bacteria so small they can only be seen through a microscope, 15
Mitosis (meye-TOH-sus), the crosswise division of one cell forming two cells, 17
  illustrated, 42
Mixed nerves, contain both sensory and motor fibers and have the ability to both send and receive messages, 53
Moist heat, sanitation and, 25
Mold, nail, is a fungus infection of the nail that is usually caused when moisture seeps between an artificial nail and the free edge of the nail, 69
Mole, is a small, brown spot on the skin. Moles range in color from tan to brown or bluish black, 82
Motor nerves, carry impulses from the brain to the muscles, 53
  move the blood vessels, 76
MSDS. See Material Safety Data Sheets (MSDS)
Muscles
  belly, is the middle part, 49
  foot, 50-51
  hand, 50
  insertion, is the part that moves, 49
  leg, lower, 50-51
  origin, is the part that does not move, 48-49
  parts of, 48-49
  stimulation of, 48
Muscular (MUS-kyoo-lahr)
  system, covers, shapes, and supports the skeleton, 44, 47-51
  tissue, contracts and moves various parts of the body, 43
Myology (meye-OL-oh-jee), is the study of the structure, functions, and diseases of the muscles, 47

Nail
  polish, dry, or pumice powder is used with the chamois buffer to add shine to the nail, 98
  acrylic,
    application procedure, 153-157
    maintenance, 162-165
    odorless, 166
    over tips/natural nails, 158-162
    post-service, 157-158
    pre-service, 153
    removal, 165
    supplies for, 152-153
  art,
    air brush and, 180
    foil, 177
    gems, 176
    holly berries, 178-179
    marbled gold, 179-180
    striping tape, 176-177
    "the sweep," 179
  bed, is the portion of skin beneath the nail body that the nail plate rests upon, 63
  biting, 68
  bleach, 98
  body, is the main part or plate of the nail that is attached to the skin at the tip of the finger, 63
  bruised, is a condition in which a clot of blood forms under the nail plate, 65
  brush, manicure and, 95
  client's needs, determining, 85
  condition of, determining, 84
  conditioner, contains moisturizes, and should be applied at night before bedtime to help prevent brittle nails and dry cuticles, 99
  cosmetics, 97-99
  discolored, is a condition in which the nails turn a variety of colors including yellow, blue, blue-grey, green, red, and purple, 65
  disorder, is a condition caused by injury to the nail or disease or imbalance in the body, 64
  disorders of, 64-71
    not serviceable by a nail technician, 69-71
    serviceable by a nail technician, 65-69
  eggshell, are thin, white, and curved over the free edge. The condition is caused by improper diet, internal disease, medication, or nervous disorders, 65
  exposing the natural, 18-19
  file, metal, manicure and, 94
  fold, also called mantle, is the deep fold of skin at the base of the nail where the nail root is embedded, 64
  free edge, is the end of the nail that extends beyond the fingertip, 63
  fungus, 18
  furrows, also known as corrugations, are long ridges that run either lengthwise or across the nail, 65-66
  golden rule of, if the nail or skin to be worked on is infected, broken, or swollen, a nail technician should not service the client, 65
  grooves, are slits or tracks in the nail bed at the sides of the nail on which the nail grows, 64
  matrix (MAY-triks), contains nerves together with lymph and blood vessels that produce nail cells and control the rate of growth of the nail, 64
  mold, 18
    is a fungus infection of the nail that is usually caused when moisture seeps between an artificial nail and the free edge of the nail, 69
    preventing, 19
  parts of, 63
  root, is where the nail growth begins. It is embedded underneath the skin at the base of the nail, 63
  shape, choosing a, 101-102
  skin surrounding the, 64
  strengthener/hardener, is applied to the natural nail before the base coat, 99
  structures of, 63-64
  tips,
    application of, 134-137
    maintenance of, 138

removal of, 138
supplies for, 133
wall, is the skin on the sides of the nail above the grooves, 64
whitener, 98
wraps,
 fabric, 145-147
 liquid, 149
 paper, 148-149
 post-service, 144
 pre-service, 141-142
 procedure, 142-144
 supplies for, 141
Natural immunity, 20
Nerve cell, is the primary structural unit of the nervous system, 53
Nerve tissue, carries messages to and from the brain, and controls and coordinates all body functions, 43
Nerves
 are long, white cords made up of fibers that carry messages to and from various parts of the body, 53, 76
 nervous system and, 52-53
 skin, 76-77
Nervous system
 brain, 52-53
 controls and coordinates the functions of all the other systems and makes them work in harmony, 44, 52
 nerves and, 53-54
 spinal cord and, 52-53
Neurology, is the branch of medicine that deals with the nervous system, 52
Neuron (NOOR-on), is the primary structural unit of the nervous system, 53
Nevus (NEE-vus)
 or birthmark, is a malformation of the skin due to abnormal pigmentation or dilated capillaries, 82
 is a brown or black stain on the nail caused by a pigmented mole that occurs on the nail, 66
No-light gel, application, 174-175
Nodules, are small tumors, 79
Non-striated muscles, are involuntary. Muscles of the stomach and intestines are non-striated, 48
Nonpathogenic (non-path-o-JEN-ik), non-disease causing, 15
Nucleus (NOO-klee-us), is made of dense protoplasm and is found in the center of the cell within the nuclear membrane, 41
Nylon fiber, is a combination of clear polish with nylon fibers. It is applied first vertically and then horizontally on the nail plate, 99

Oil glands, secrete an oily substance, called sebum, 77-78
Onychatrophia (on-i-kah-TROH-fee-ah), also known as atrophy is the wasting away of the nail, 66
Onychauxis (on-i-KIK-sis), is the overgrowth of nails, 66-67
Onychia (on-NIK-ee-ah), is an inflammation somewhere in the nail, 69
Onychocryptosis (on-i-koh-krip-TOH-sis), the nail grows into the sides of the tissue around the nail, 67
Onychogryphosis (on-i-koh-greye-FOH-sis), is a condition in which the nail curvature is increased and enlarged, 69
Onycholysis (on-i-KOL-i-sis), is a condition in which the nail loosens from the nail bed, beginning usually at the free edge and continuing to the lunula, but does not come off, 70
Onychomycosis (oni-koh-meye-KOH-sis), tinea unguim (TIN-ee-ah Un-gwee-um), is an infectious disease caused by a fungus (vegetable parasite), 69-70
Onychophagy (on-i-KOH-fa-jee), is the medical term for nails that have been bitten enough to become deformed, 67
Onychoptosis (on-i-kop-TOH-sis), is a condition in which part or all of the nail sheds periodically and falls off the finger, 70
Onychorrhexis (on-i-kohr-RED-sis), refers to split or brittle nails that also have a series of lengthwise ridges, 68
Opponent muscles, are located in the palm of the hand and act to bring the thumb toward the fingers, allowing the grasping action of the hands, 50
Orangewood stick, manicure and, 94
Organs, body, 43

Paper wraps, 148-149
Papillae (pa-PIL-e), little cone-like projections that extend upward into the epidermis, 76
Papillary (PA-pil-ah-ry) layer, lies directly under the epidermis and contains the papillae, 76
Papule (PAP-chool), is a small pimple that does not contain fluid, but can develop pus, 79
Parasites (PAR-ah-syts), are multicelled animal or vegetable organisms, 19
Paronychia (par-oh-NIK-ee-ah), is a bacterial inflammation of the tissue around the nail, 70-71
Paronychium (par-oh-NIK-ee-um), is the part of the skin that surrounds the entire nail area, 64
Patella (pah-TEL-lah), also called the accessory bone, forms the knee cap, 46
Pathogenic (path-o-JEN-ik), disease causing, 15
Pedicure
 post-service, 126-127
 pre-service for, 122-123
 procedure, 123-126
 supplies for, 121-122
Pericardium (per-i-KAHR-dee-um), the sack in which the heart is enclosed, 55
Peripheral (pe-RIF-er-al) nervous system, is made up of the sensory and motor nerve fibers that extend from the brain and spinal cord and are distributed to all parts of the body, 52
Peroneus
 brevis (per-oh-NEE-us BREV-us), originates on the lower surface of the fibula. It bends the foot down and out, 51
 longus (per-oh-NEE-us LONG-us), covers the outer side of the calf and inverts the foot and turns it outward, 51
Personal records, keeping, 185
Phalanges (fl-LAN-jeez)
 foot, are similar to the finger bones, 47
 finger, in each finger and two in the thumb, totaling fourteen bones, 46
Pharynx (FAR-ingks), 60
Pivot (PIH-vut) joints, one bone turns on another bone, 45
Plasma, is the fluid part of the blood, in which the red and white blood cells and blood platelets flow, 57
Plastic bags, manicure and, 97
Polish
 application, types of, 107-108
 remover, 98
Popliteal (pop-lih-TEE-ul) artery, divides into two separate arteries in supplying blood to the lower leg, 58
Posterior tibial artery, is located in the lower leg, 58
Products, selling, 191-195
Pronator (PRO-nay-tor), turns the hands inward, so the palm faces downward, 49
Protein hardener, is a combination of clear polish and protein, such as collagen, 99
Protoplasm (PROH-toh-plaz-em), is a colorless, jellylike substance that contains food elements such as protein, fat, carbohydrates, and mineral salts, 41

Psoriasis (so-REYE-a-sis), is a chronic inflammation with round, dry patches covered with coarse silvery scales, 80

Pterygium (te-RIJ-ee-um), describes the common condition of the forward growth of the cuticle on the nail, 68

Pulmonary (PUL-mo-ner-ee), circulation, is the blood circulation that goes from the heart to the lungs to be purified, 56

Pumice (PUM-is) powder, or dry nail polish is used with the chamois buffer to add shine to the nail, 98

Pusher, steel, manicure and, 94

Pustule (PUS-chool), is a lump on the skin with an inflamed base and a head containing pus, 79

Pyrogenic granuloma, is a severe inflammation of the nail in which a lump of red tissue grows up from the nail bed to the nail plate, 71

Quaternary ammonium (QUAT-er-nery a-MOHN-ee-um) compounds, are a broad range of chemical agents available under different trade and chemical names, in liquid and tablet form, 27

Radial (RAY-dee-al)
   artery, main artery supplying blood to the arm and hand, 57
   nerve, and its branches supply the thumb side of the arm and the back of the hand, 53

Radius (RAY-dee-us), is the small bone in the forearm on the same side as the thumb, 45

Receptors, are sensory nerve endings located near the surface of the skin, 53

Reconditioning hot oil manicure and, 109-110
   pre-service, 110
   procedure, 110-111

Records
   business, 186
   inventory, 187
   personal, 185
   service, 187

Red corpuscles (KOR-pus-els), blood cells which carry oxygen to the cells, 57

Reflex, is an automatic response to a stimulus that involves the transmission of an impulse from a sensory receptor along an afferent nerve to the spinal cord, and a responsive impulse along an efferent neuron to a muscle, causing a reaction, 53

Reproductive system, enables human beings to reproduce, 44

Respiratory (RES-pi-rah-toh-ree) system
   is situated within the chest cavity, which is protected on both sides of the ribs, 60
   supplies oxygen to the body, 44

Reticular (re-TIK-u-lar) layer, contains fat cells, blood and lymph vessels, sweat and oil glands, and hair follicles, 76

Rickettsia (rik-ET-see-ah), are much smaller organisms than bacteria, but larger than viruses. They cause typhus and Rocky Mountain spotted fever and are carried by ticks, fleas, and lice, 19

Right
   atrium (AY-tree-um), one of the upper, thin-walled chambers of the heart, 56
   ventricle (VEN-tri-kel), one of the lower, thick-walled chambers of the heart, 56

Ringworm (tinea), of the hand is a highly contagious disease caused by a fungus, 81

Salon
   advertising, 189

booking appointments, 187-188, 195
business decisions concerning, 184
full-service, 183
nails-only, 183-184
payment collection, 189
records,
   business, 186
   inventory, 187
   keeping personal, 185
   service, 187
safety in, 33-38

Sanitation
   chemical agents for, 25
   equipment used in, 25-26
   methods of, 24
   physical agents for, 25
   pre-service procedure of, 29
   solutions, making, 26-27

Saphenous (sa-FEEN-us) nerve, supplies impulses to the skin of the inner side of the leg and foot, 54

Saprophyte (SAP-rop-fyt), bacteria that feed on dead matter and cause decay, 15

Scales, skin, are produced during shedding of the epidermis, 79

Scapula (SKAP-yoo-lah), forms the shoulder, 45

Scar, is a light-colored, slightly raised mark on the skin formed after an injury or lesion of the skin has healed, 79

Sealer, is a colorless polish, is applied over colored polish to prevent chipping and add a shine to the finished nail, 99

Sebaceous (si-BAY-shus) glands, secrete an oily substance, called sebum, 77-78

Secretory (se-KREET-e-ree) nerves, are the nerves of the sweat and oil glands, 77

Sensory nerves
   are found in the papillary layer of the dermis, give the skin sense of touch, 76-77
   carry impulses or messages from sense organs to the brain, 53

Service records, 187
   client's, 88

Shoulder, muscles of, 49

Skeletal system
   is the physical foundation or framework of the body. The bones of the skeletal system serve as a means of protection, support, and locomotion, 44
   described, 44-47

Skin
   broken, occurs when the epidermis is cut or torn, exposing the deeper layers of the skin, 78
   golden rule of, if the nail or skin to be work on is infected, broken, or swollen, a nail technician should not service the client, 65, 78
   client's needs, determining, 85
   condition of, determining, 84
   diagram of, 75
   dips, 80
   disorders of, 78-81
   elasticity of, 78
   function of, 73-74
   glands of, 77-78
   infected, will show evidence of pus, 78
   infections of, 81
   inflamed, is red, sore, and swollen, 78
   inflammations of, 80
   lesion (LEE-zhun), is a structural change in tissue caused by injury or disease, 79
   lesions of, 79
   nerves of, 76-77
   nourishment of, 76

pigmentation of, 81-82
  raised, is a symptom of a variety of skin conditions some of which are lesions, 78
  structure of, 74-76
Soap, antibacterial, 97
Sodium hypochlorite (SOH-di-um hy-po-CHLOR-ite), or household bleach is a sanitizing agent now used because of the threat of the HIV virus, 28
Soleus (SO-lee-us), originates at the upper portion of the fibula and bends the foot down, 51
Spatula, manicure and, 97
Spinal cord, nervous system and, 52-53
Spirilla (spi-RIL-a), are spiral or corkscrew-shaped bacteria that include spirochetal organisms, 16
Stain, is an abnormal discoloration that remains after moles, freckles, or liver spots disappear, or after certain diseases, 79
Staphylococci (staf-i-lo-KOK-si), grow in clusters and are present in local infections, 16
Steaming, sanitation and, 25
Steel pusher, manicure and, 94
Stomach, digest food, 43
Stratum
  corneum (STRAT-um KOHR-nee-um), also called the horny layer, which consists of tightly packed, scale like cells that are continually shed and replaced, 75
  germinativum (STRAT-um jur-mi-nah-TIV-um), is composed of several layers of differently shaped cells, 75
  granulosum (STRAT-um gran-yoo-LOH-sum) consists of cells that look like granules, 75
  lucidum (STRAT-um LOO-si-dum), is a small layer of clear cells that light can pass through, 75
Striated (STRY-ate-id) muscles, are voluntary muscles that you can move whenever you want, 47
Striping tape, nail art and, 176-177
Styptic (STIP-tik) powder, is used to contract the skin to stop minor bleeding that may occur during a manicure, 97
Subcutaneous tissue, is made up of fatty tissue known as adipose, 76
Sudoriferous (su-dohr-IF-er-us) glands, sweat glands that regulate body temperature and eliminate waste products through perspiration, 77
Superficial peroneal nerve, passes downward in front of the fibula and supplies impulses to the skin of the foot and toes, 54
Supinator (SUE-pi-nay-tor), turns the hand outward so the palm faces upward, 49
Supply tray, manicure and, 94
Sural nerve, supplies impulses to the outer side and back of the foot and leg, 54
Sweat pore, is a small opening in the skin surface from which the sweat gland eliminates waste, 77
Synovial (sy-NOV-ee-al) fluid, is the lubrication that prevents friction at the joints where bones meet, 45
Systemic circulation, is the blood circulation from the heart throughout the body and back again to the heart, 56
Systems, body, 44

Tactile corpuscles (TAK-til KOR-puh-sils), are nerve endings, 76
Tan, is the darkening of the skin caused by exposure to the ultraviolet rays of the sun, 82
Tarsal (TAR-sul) bones, the seven bones that make up the ankle, 46
Tenth cranial nerve, regulates the heartbeat, 55
Tibia (TIB-ee-ah), is the larger of the two bones that form the leg below the knee, 46
Tibial (TIB-ee-al) nerve, located in the thigh, passes behind the knee. It subdivides and supplies impulses to the knee, the muscles of the calf, the skin of the leg, and the sole, heel, and underside of the toes, 54
Tibialis anterior (tib-ee-AHL-is an-TEHR-ee-ohr), covers the front of the shin. It bends the foot upward and inward, 51
Tinea pedis (TIN-ee-ah PEH-dus), also known as athlete's foot or ringworm of the foot, is a fungus infection of the foot, 81
Tissues, described, 43
Top coat, is a colorless polish, is applied over colored polish to prevent chipping and add a shine to the finished nail, 99
Towels, manicure and, 97
Triceps, are muscles that cover the entire back of the upper arm and extend the forearm forward, 49
Tubercle (TOO-ber-kyool), is a solid lump larger than a papule. It varies in size from a pea to a hickory nut, 79
Tumor, is an abnormal cell mass that varies in size, shape, and color, 79
Tweezers, manicure and, 95

Ulcer, is an open lesion on the skin or mucous membrane of the body, 80
Ulna (UL-nah), is the large bone on the small-finger side of the forearm, 45
Ulnar (UL-nar)
  artery, main artery supplying blood to the arm and hand, 57
  nerve, and its branches supply the small finger side of the arm and the palm of the hand, 53
Ultraviolet ray
  electrical sanitizer, is used to keep implements clean until ready for use, 26
  sanitation and, 25

Vagus (VAY-gus) nerve, regulates the heartbeat, 55
Valves, heart, allow the blood to flow in only one direction, 56
Vascular (VAS-kyoo-lahr) system, controls the steady circulation of the blood through the body by means of the heart and blood vessels, 55
Veins, carry blood that lacks oxygen from the capillaries back to the heart. They are thin-walled blood vessels that are less elastic than arteries. They contain cuplike valves to prevent backflow. Veins are closer to the surface of the body than arteries are, 56
Ventricle (VEN-tri-kel), the two lower, thick-walled chambers of the heart, 56
Vesicle (VES-i-kell), is a blister containing clear fluid, 80
Viruses, are pathogenic agents that are many times smaller than bacteria, 17
Vitiligo (vit-l-EYE-go), is an acquired form of leucoderma that affects the skin or hair, 82

Water manicure
  post-service, 108
  pre-service, 102-103
  procedure, 103-108
Wet sanitizer, any glass receptacle that is large enough to hold disinfectant solution and a submerged, or completely covered implement, 25-26
Wheals (HWEELS), or hives are swollen, itchy bumps on the skin that last for several hours, 80
White corpuscles, blood cells that perform the function of destroying disease-causing germs, 57